A PLUME BOOK

HYPOCHONDRIA CAN KILL

JOHN NAISH writes for *The Times* in London. He is a t'ai chi–practicing vegetarian who enjoys rock music and fast motorcycles.

Hypochondria Can kill

JOHN NAISH

A PLUME BOOK

PLUME
Published by Penguin Group
Penguin Group (USA) Inc., 375 Hudson Street,
New York, New York 10014, U.S.A.
Penguin Group (Canada), 90 Eglinton Avenue East, Suite 700, Toronto,
Ontario, Canada M4P 2Y3 (a division of Pearson Penguin Canada Inc.)
Penguin Books Ltd., 80 Strand, London WC2R 0RL, England
Penguin Ireland, 25 St. Stephen's Green, Dublin 2, Ireland
(a division of Penguin Books Ltd.)
Penguin Group (Australia), 250 Camberwell Road, Camberwell,
Victoria 3124, Australia (a division of Pearson Australia Group Pty. Ltd.)
Penguin Books India Pvt. Ltd., 11 Community Centre, Panchsheel Park,
New Delhi – 110 017, India
Penguin Books (NZ), cnr Airborne and Rosedale Roads, Albany,
Auckland 1310, New Zealand (a division of Pearson New Zealand Ltd.)
Penguin Books (South Africa) (Pty.) Ltd., 24 Sturdee Avenue, Rosebank,
Johannesburg 2196, South Africa

Penguin Books Ltd., Registered Offices: 80 Strand,
London WC2R 0RL, England

First published by Plume, a member of Penguin Group (USA) Inc.

First Printing, November 2005

10   9   8   7   6   5   4   3   2   1

Copyright © John Naish, 2005
All rights reserved

℗ REGISTERED TRADEMARK—MARCA REGISTRADA

CIP data is available.
ISBN 0-452-28688-3

Printed in the United States of America
Set in Adobe Garamond

Contents

Introduction

Let's invent a new illness. Let's call it Modern Hypochondria Syndrome (MHS). The symptoms? Gnawing health anxiety; fascination for new diseases; an impulse to throw cash at costly therapies; excessive use of words such as "well-being" and "nutrient." Risk factors: living in a comfortably rich nation and having a lack of real threats to fret about. We've just created MHS, a new and worrying social disease. Easy.

Well, it was no harder than inventing Pleasure Deficiency Syndrome, which a survey of 2,000 people warned is sweeping the Western world. In November 2003 the survey, by the internet pollsters YouGov, quoted psychologist Dr. Linda Papadopoulos claiming that victims of the syndrome suffer tiredness, boredom with work, and lethargy. "There is evidence that people are malfunctioning because they are not enjoying enough pleasure on a regular basis to be healthy happy people," she says.

If that doesn't get you throwing your arms about in panic, then consider Celebrity Worship Syndrome (CWS), which apparently affects one in three Britons and is "borderline pathological" in severe cases. CWS victims can be "impulsive, troublesome and insensitive," says a report of the study in the *Journal of Nervous and Mental Disease* (2003, 191; 1:25). So watch out, or one day you might wake up to find yourself stalking a daytime-TV game-show host.

CWS is hardly the Fifth Horseman. War, Plague, Famine, Death, and Celebrity Worship Syndrome. But such silly sicknesses are becoming epidemic. The developed world is safer than ever, but new "illnesses" continually emerge to keep doctors, therapists, and drug companies hale and hearty. Our appetite for the latest threat seems insatiable.

We all, to some extent, carry the germs of hypochondria. We evolved mild doses of it as a survival tool. Our cavepersons' brains are hardwired to obsess about threats. We relish tales of strange and deadly illness like winter-nights' horror stories. Thanks to modern sanitation and medicine, those dangers are now no longer anywhere near so real. But at the same time, civilization has given us much more time, cash, and energy to spend fixating on sickness. So while the Western world has enjoyed a huge drop in mortal illnesses, it has witnessed a leap in new diagnoses.

How many people (psychopaths apart) do you know who, deep down, are cheerfully convinced that there is absolutely nothing wrong with them? I bet that if you were to put on a pair of white overalls, drive an ambulance-type vehicle along the main street, pull up next to any pedestrian, leap out and say, "Get in, we've found out what's wrong with you," most would willingly be helped limply into the back.

Many doctors worry about the trend to prescribe ever-more new drugs and treatments for an ever-growing list of new illnesses. Norman M. Hadler, a professor of medicine at North Carolina University and author of the 2004 book, *The Last Well Person: How to Stay Well Despite the Health-Care System,* says overmedicalization is a threat to health, turning the United States into a nation of worried well people who cannot cope with life's everyday trials and twinges. A poll of doctors on the top "non-diseases" that are being redefined as medical conditions was held in the *British Medical Journal* (2002; 324:7334). In first place was aging, followed by work, boredom, and bags under the eyes. Others included baldness, freckles, ugliness, jet lag, shortness, nail biting, bad breath, insomnia, and hairiness.

But many other doctors are keen to discover, or invent, new illnesses for us. It gets them published in the profession's fast-expanding body of story-hungry research journals. If their new disease is scary enough—or sexy enough—it might get their name in the newspapers. And if they can specialize in treating their new illness, it could make them a lot of money.

The old demon, money, lurks behind much hypochondria. The pharmaceutical industry needs new plagues as badly as the rest of us. If it cured everything, commercial growth would grind to a shareholder-sickening halt. The industry thrives by providing cures—though companies have found it is a cute trick to invent cures for diseases that don't quite exist. They, after all, are much easier to tackle.

The Royal College of General Practitioners warned the U.K. government in August 2004 that drug companies' classification of conditions such as hypertension and depression as abnormal are "not in the interests of patients and serve only to reward the industry itself." The College's Dr. Maureen Baker told Parliament: "It is always difficult to draw a simple line between what is normal and what is an illness, but it is in the interest of the pharmaceutical industry to draw a line which includes as large a population as possible within the 'ill' category. The bigger this group is the more drugs they can sell."

Thus, mere conditions get juiced up into diseases by drug companies' highly paid public-relations departments, and rare illnesses are pushed as being on the increase. Everyday traits such as shyness grow into sicknesses. Roche developed the drug Mannerix to treat "social phobia," and claimed that 1 million Australians suffered from it. But the company could not initially find enough sufferers for clinical trials. That was a few years back. Now, social phobia is becoming accepted as a condition. Pfizer markets the drug Zoloft in America as a cure for Social Anxiety Disorder. Yep, SAD.

New technology has boosted our lust for scary info about illnesses. Health is now the second most popular internet search topic, after pornography. Doctors call it *cyberchondria.* People with minor everyday snuffles Google their symptoms and strike an oozing seam of illness. Indigestion, say the websites, could be stomach cancer, headaches might be a brain tumor, those pins and needles could mean multiple sclerosis.

The final culprits in stoking up modern hypochondria are people like me, who work in the information industry. Readers want to pore over newly discovered threats to their health and sanity, and journalists are perfectly happy to oblige—often by rewriting drug companies' overblown press releases with a cynically uncritical eye.

Two community health experts complained in the *British Medical Journal* on February 28, 2004, that in the previous month alone they had read newspaper reports about studies that "proved" moving to the countryside, drinking wine, or discussing your relationship problems in bed can improve sexual problems. They also read that owning a pet helps you recover more quickly from illness, testosterone causes unsafe sex, and text messaging is good for your mental health.

But it's all a load of public-relations eyewash, they say: "PR companies have big budgets to promote their research, to the exclusion of more reliable, ethical work. Often the PR company has decided on the outcome way before the study begins. Because PR survey results are presented as startling, journalists may see a good headline, a light story, or a way of meeting a looming deadline."

The Oxford-based Social Issues Research Centre recently attacked the media's habit of raising false hopes by publicizing medical breakthroughs that do not exist. "There must come a time when excessive, unfounded hyping, often amounting to nothing more than cruel hoaxes, is curtailed," it says. Some hope. Who wants a bunch of complicated stats and facts to ruin a good yarn?

But in spite of all this, we should not feel bad about our modern-day mass neuroses. That could cause an epidemic of Hyperchondriasis Denial Syndrome to afflict millions of highly vulnerable health addicts. Instead, we should take the chance to celebrate the masterpiece of human creativity that is hypochondria.

What follows is the result of my squirreling hundreds of daft, disturbing, rare, strange, spurious, wacko, and sometimes plain disgusting health research reports into a desk drawer while spending the past decade as a health journalist. From this medical mulch has grown a monument to the hypochondriacal human condition.

It is also a tribute to hard work—in the shape of druggists' hype, quacks' creativity, researchers' resourcefulness, journalists' craven sensationalism—and, of course, the sheer paranoid pleasure that we take in swallowing it all on a daily basis.

Taken en masse, this overdose of doom might even be sufficient to make right-thinking people decide to give up obsessing about their health and instead get on with living a neurosis-free life in the safest era that humanity has ever known. Now that, ultimately, would be a massive achievement for medical science.

Important Note

Clinical studies show that hypochondria can kill (see page 21)—and that people who fret are more likely to develop cancer and Alzheimer's disease (page 134). Please remember at all times to not let any of the information in this book worry you. Try taking it all with a pinch of salt. Not too much salt, mind you.

References explained: Want to know more (or just plain don't believe it)? Most entries are referenced from medical journals. The system is this: an entry such as (2002, 15; 167:1104) translates as (year, volume; issue number:page number). Volume numbers are sometimes not given.

Hypochondria Can kill

HOME COMFORTS

For hypochondria begins at home . . .

Telephone Stroke

Look out chatterboxes: if you love to
spend hours on the phone, there's a risk
of giving yourself a debilitating stroke,
warns the *Canadian Medical Association Journal* (2002, 10; 167:1104).

Dr. Malvinder Parmar, the medical
director of Timmins and District
Hospital in Northern Ontario, says he
discovered "telephone stroke" after examining a sixty-three-year-old man who had developed
slurred speech, unsteadiness, and weakness on his left
side right after finishing a fifty-six-minute phone call.

He had suffered an obstruction of his bloodflow,
which Dr. Parmar says was most probably caused by the
compression of a crucial artery during the phone call,
when the victim kept his head bent to the right side. The
doctor says that to avoid such an injury, you should play
it safe and change sides often, or think about using a
hands-free set at home. Or just talk less.

Dr. Parmar adds telephone stroke to medicine's list of
similar conditions caused by neck-benders such as chiro-
practic manipulation, protracted dental work, X-ray po-
sitioning and . . .

Beauty Parlor Syndrome

Vanity can come at a crippling price, and not only at the make-up counter. Beauty parlor syndrome was identified by Michael Weintraub of the New York Medical College, Valhalla. He was alerted to the perils of keeping up appearances after seeing five female patients admitted to the hospital suffering from strokes that occurred after they had gone for a hairdo.

The women, from ages fifty-four to eighty-four, left the parlors with a range of strokelike symptoms, from vertigo to partial paralysis. Weintraub believes they suffered injuries to the arteries carrying blood to the brain when their heads were stretched backward over the hairdressers' sinks. He sent a message to parlor-owners in the *Journal of the American Medical Association* (1993, 269; 16:2086): go easy on older clients.

Handkerchief of Grief

Should Kleenex carry a health warning? Vigorous nose-blowing can in rare cases create a blast of internal pressure so powerful it will crack your orbit, the bony cavity in which the eye sits. And that may lead to serious trouble, doctors warn.

Hard nose-blowing can force air through a fractured eye socket into the skull, where it could cause emphysema—air trapped in tissues where air should not be, say doctors at Birmingham City Hospital, England. They report how one twenty-year-old woman managed to blast so much air through her broken eye socket that it ended up in her chest cavity, causing significant pain, in the *Journal of Laryngology & Otology* (2003, 117; 2:141).

Overenthusiastic honking can potentially cause blindness, because of the possible effects of air pressure and infection, warn doctors at Craigavon Area Hospital, Northern Ireland, in the same publication (2001, 115; 4:319). More comfortingly, though, they say that often the fracture will spontaneously repair itself in around two weeks.

Deafening Blow

It is not only the eyes and chest that are imperiled by vigorous blowing. Japanese doctors from Kawanishi Municipal Hospital report how one fifty-five-year-old man suffered blower's deafness in both ears after a good old blast into his handkerchief. He gradually developed vertigo and then his left eyeball started oscillating. The eye trouble and vertigo cleared up, but a year later his hearing had not improved, says the case study in the *Nippon Jibiinkoka Gakkai Kaiho* (1997, 100; 11:1375). The medics say the damage was caused by the patient overpressurizing his inner ears.

Some people just ask for trouble, though. German doctors report in *Laryngorhinootologie* (1992, 71; 9:485) how another patient achieved much the same injury by trying to inflate a party balloon with his nose.

FASHION VICTIMS

Those trousers a bit snug? Waddling about in skin-tight slacks not only makes you look ridiculous, it could also land you in dire straits. Dr. Octavio Bessa, of Stanford, Connecticut, reports how he kept seeing patients with mystery stomach pains that modern medical diagnostics could not explain.

He realized that the patients had recently put on weight, but had not invested in larger clothes. "I noticed that the difference between these patients' abdominal girth measurement and pants size is usually 7.5 cm (3 in.). All the symptoms disappear after the use of suspenders and change in pants size," he says in the *Archives of Internal Medicine* (1993, 153; 11:1396). "I have coined this the tight pants syndrome."

Dr. Deborah Allen of the Indiana University School of Medicine, Indianapolis, replied to Bessa, saying that overweight patients often show signs of hiatus hernias which disappear under examination—because they have removed the offending trousers.

Trucker's Trouser

Similar problems appear among those notorious fashion victims—truck drivers. "Most of them are obese and wear tight-fitting denims," says Dr. J. R. Boyce of the University of Alabama in Birmingham. He reports in the *Journal of the American Medical Association* (1984, 251; 12:1553) that, "A number of truck drivers who consented to wearing loose-fitting, albeit less fashionable, trousers had notable improvement of their symptoms."

Hipster Hell

Still more trouser-related trauma has been blamed on hiphugger pants coming back into fashion. These can cause mystery burning sensations in the thighs.

Malvinder Parmar, the medical director at Timmins and District Hospital, Northern Ontario, Canada, says he encountered three "mildly obese young women" between the ages of twenty-two and thirty-five, who had worn tight low-rise pants over the previous six to eight months. All had symptoms of tingling or burning sensations on the side of the thigh.

One of the women was becoming convinced she had multiple sclerosis and wanted an MRI scan, but Parmar decided that pressure on her lateral femoral cutaneous nerve was the problem, and her hiphuggers were the cause. His prescription, in the *Canadian Medical Association Journal* (2003, 168; 1:16), was for her to wear loose-fitting dresses.

Lingerie Department

The G-string, the modern way to avoid the dreaded visible panty line, is blamed for causing health troubles, too. The skimpy panties have been fingered for causing nasty chronic infections. The *Patient's Encyclopedia of Cystitis* warns that many designs have hard seams that can irritate the vaginal area and the string can transfer bacteria from the bottom.

That other modern lingerie phenomenon, the push-up bra, has also been criticized by experts who claim that constricting brassieres can cause back pain. Medical anthropologist Sydney Singer claims that tight bras may cause congestion in the lymph nodes and thus stop the body from flushing out toxins, reports the *Kansas City Star* (June 26, 1995). He argues that breast cancer is a problem only among cultures where women wear bras. The British School of Osteopathy doesn't like push-up bras either. It says they may be linked to a wide range of health problems such as breathing difficulties and spinal pain, and even side effects such as constipation and irritable bowel syndrome.

UNDONE BY FLIES

The males of the species live in peril of their clothes, too. How many guys have been undone by their flies? Researchers can only guess that most men have suffered penile zip injury. Most often it is a trauma suffered in childhood—just one of life's more painful little lessons. Scottish emergency-room consultants report in *Injury* (1994, 25; 1:59) that one in every four thousand new patients is a trouser-trapped child.

But plenty of men forget that important formative lesson, says Richard Hockey, a data analyst at Australia's Queensland Injury Surveillance Unit. He found that trapped genitals are far and away the leading cause of clothing-related injury when he analyzed emergency department statistics from 1998 to 2001.

"People probably try to treat themselves first. The embarrassment factor might put you off seeking help as long as possible," he says in the *Medical Post* (October 8, 2002). "Maybe it is seasonal. In the hotter weather, anecdotally, people are going without underpants."

Medical science is split on the best course of action. New York doctors in *Pediatric Emergency Care* (1993, 9; 2:90) suggest you can free fly-trapped men by pouring mineral oil over the zipper, while across the Atlantic, researchers in *European Urology* (1981, 7; 6:365) suggest cutting across the zipper where it has pinched the foreskin. Others suggest a rapid yank downward should do the trick.

Old-fashioned button flies might be the best long-term answer.

Wallet Warning

One further cause of male trouser trauma: Elmar Lutz of St. Mary's Hospital, New Jersey, reports two cases of patients suffering mysterious painful thighs and lower backs—one example lasted fourteen months, the other eight years. Slipped discs had been investigated, chiropractors visited, but to no avail.

The answer, Lutz realized, is the previously unknown danger of sitting on a fat wallet for great lengths of time. One patient's wallet was more than one-inch thick and contained a small library of credit cards.

In each case, credit card sciatica was cured by "the simple procedure of a walletectomy"—that is, taking it out of the patient's pocket, says Lutz in the *Journal of the American Medical Association* (1978, 240; 8:738). Relief was "fairly immediate."

"I have encountered several other cases over the years and this tends to indicate that the problem is more common than realized," he says. "If unrelieved, it could lead eventually to more severe neurovascular dysfunction and nerve injury."

Money Worries?

If you have an aversion to meeting the bank manager, it might not simply come down to the perilous state of your finances. You could have a real illness. Researchers at Cambridge University, England, claim to have discovered a psychological condition they call *financial phobia*. They say that it affects more than 9 million people in Britain alone.

Sufferers become seized with anxiety, guilt, or boredom when confronted with the need to manage their money. They resort to avoidance techniques such as not checking bank balances and, in extreme cases, throwing away unopened statements. Nearly half of a sample of a thousand otherwise well-adjusted people polled experienced a racing heart when faced with managing money, 15 percent said they felt immobilized, 12 percent felt physically ill, and 11 percent went dizzy.

Brendan Burchell, a senior lecturer in social and political sciences, says in *The Guardian* (January 27, 2003) that financial phobia affects 20 percent of the population, particularly women and young people. Nearly a third of those asked said they would rather visit the dentist than sit down with a bank statement.

Biblio-piles

Please don't leave this book in the bathroom. Reading while sitting on the toilet can give you hemorrhoids, warns an article in the *Lancet* (1989, 1; 8628:54). Doctors at the John Radcliffe Hospital, Oxford, United Kingdom, compared the habits of one hundred people suffering from hemorrhoids with one hundred unaffected people and found that a much larger proportion of the group suffering from hemorrhoids read in the bathroom. Reading in itself is not bad for you, but sitting in the restroom for long periods causes undue pressure on your bottom, say the Oxford doctors.

Diary Danger

Literature is not only dangerous in the lavatory: memoir-keeping can cause misery, too. Writing down your secret fears and woes might sound therapeutic, but in fact, keeping a regular diary is bad for your health, warn psychologists. They say diarists are more likely than non-diarists to suffer from headaches, aches, pains, and feeling run-down.

"We expected diary keepers to have some benefit, or to be the same, but they were worse off," Elaine Duncan of the Glasgow Caledonian University told the British Psychology Society's annual conference in Edinburgh, Scotland (September 8, 2004).

She and a colleague studied ninety-four regular diarists and compared their health with forty-one non-diarists. The diary-writers scored much worse on health measures than the non-diarists. People who reread their diaries reported greater levels of anxiety and distress. Worst affected of all were those who had written about trauma.

"You're probably much better off if you don't write anything at all," says Duncan.

HOUSEWORK MASSACRES MEN

DIY (Do It Yourself) might better be spelled DYI—Do Yourself In—if we are to believe figures showing that men have a ten-times higher risk of death per minute spent doing home maintenance than women, and even manage a four-times greater risk of suffering a fatality when performing simple "housework."

The statistics, culled from coroners' files in Australia over a three-year period, show what dangerous places homes can be if you are male. Men represent 83 percent of home-death victims. The study found that the most common items involved in deaths were ladders (18 percent), collapsing car jacks (7 percent), and portable electric cables (5 percent). Many of the deaths were remarkably similar, say the researchers in the journal *Injury Prevention* (2003, 9; 1:15).

They were

"Persons (usually male) performing maintenance on cars which were inadequately jacked up and which rolled or fell on them, causing death through crush asphyxia or head injuries.

"Persons (usually male) performing maintenance on the home with faulty equipment or without ensuring that the relevant electrical circuits had been isolated.

"Persons (usually male) killed in fires started as a result of leaving the stove turned on after cooking or leaving something cooking while they fell asleep."

Play safe, men. Get a woman to do it.

It's a Jungle Out There

More than four hundred thousand Americans are treated in emergency rooms for injuries received from power lawn and garden equipment, estimates the U.S. Product Safety Commission. The *Chicago Tribune* (June 7, 2002) reports that the most common tool involved in lawn-care injuries is the ride-on mower. More than twenty-five thousand Americans are hurt and seventy-five killed every year by one.

On the other side of the Atlantic, the UK Home Accident Surveillance Statistics (2000) determined that the following gardening tools and equipment are most frequently involved in personal injuries:

Lawn mowers
Pruning shears
Hedge trimmers
Spades, shovels, and garden forks
Saws
Stepladders and ladders
Edgers

That's just the obvious stuff. More than one thousand people a year in Britain are injured by wheelbarrows. And about four hundred manage to have an accident involving a trowel.

Dishcloth Disease

That innocent-looking dishcloth could be wiping you out. Charles Gerba and his team at Arizona University in

Tucson inspected dishcloths across the United States and concluded that they are making countless people ill. The microbiologists collected dishcloths and sponges from one hundred homes in each of five big cities, and found that some sort of pathogen lurked in 70 percent of them. Twenty percent harbored salmonella and staphylococcus, the most common causes of food-borne illness in America, Gerba says in *New Scientist* (September 2, 1995).

A study covered by the International Scientific Forum on Home Hygiene says 84 percent of dishcloths are contaminated with the food-poisoning bacterium listeria. The Forum says you can get up to 1 million bacteria on your hands just by wringing out an infected sponge or dishrag.

Don't Touch That Doorknob

One door handle contaminated with harmful bacteria or viruses can infect at least the first fourteen people who touch it, according to German researchers in the *Journal of Hospital Infection* (2000; 46:61). That may be enough to cause household panic, because doorknobs, along with bathroom taps, toilet flushes, and soap dispensers, are the most common ways you can pick up viral contamination passed on by someone who didn't wash their hands after using the bathroom, according to a 2001 study for *Social Science and Medicine*.

There is apparently no escape: simply flushing the toilet after an episode of diarrhea can infect the toilet seat, lid, and surrounding air with infectious bacteria that may hang around in the toilet water for up to fifty days, reports the *Journal of Applied Microbiology* (2000; 89:137).

OR MAYBE WE SHOULD GET DIRTY?

Then again, there's the hygiene hypothesis, which argues that more and more children are developing asthma because they have not been exposed to dirt and bacteria early on. This is based on studies such as one in the *Deutsch Medical Wochenschreib* (2000, 125; 31–32:923), which followed thirteen hundred children for sixteen years and concluded that those brought up on farms had a much lower incidence of asthma than infants raised in fastidiously clean urban homes.

The scientists suspect that the lack of "environmental insults" deprive the urban children's immune systems of the early stimuli that encourage them to develop fully. The lack of exposure to our natural messy environment may mean they have persnickety defenses that can't tell the difference between threatening substances and harmless ones.

Cleaner Misdemeanor

Or maybe it's the cleaning fluids at fault. A report in *Thorax* (2004; 59:756) warns that domestic solvents and cleaning products may themselves increase the risk of childhood asthma. The researchers studied 192 preschool-age children at a hospital in Perth, Australia. They were tested for allergies and their homes checked for levels of volatile organic compounds (VOCs) of the type found in common domestic cleaning products, polishes, and fresheners.

The children exposed to above-average levels of VOCs

were four times more likely to have asthma than those who were not, say the study's authors, from Perth's Curtin University of Technology. The VOC levels did not, however, exceed maximum limits recommended by Western governments.

Dr. Imtiaz Ahmad, senior lecturer in physical chemistry at Britain's Anglia Polytechnic University, claims in the report *Chemicals Uncovered*, published in August 2004, that many popular household cleaners contain undisclosed amounts of potentially dangerous chemicals, such as alkyl phenoxy polyethoxy ethanols that are "known to accelerate growth in breast cancer cells"; butyl cellosolve, "a neurotoxin which represses the nervous system"; and crystalline silica, "a known carcinogenic, [which] also adversely affects the eyes, skin, and lungs."

Prolonged exposure to these neurotoxins can also cause suppression of the nervous system, warns Ahmad. Though one should note that her report is being used by a commercial company called BioCare—to promote a new range of "100 percent natural" home-cleaning products.

Toothbrush Terror

Cleaning the house is not the only home hazard. Cleaning yourself can result in a nasty injury. Over a twelve-month period, an estimated 2,489 people managed to hurt themselves brushing their teeth, say researchers from the U.S. Food and Drug Administration. Officially the mishaps, culled from hospital records between 1999 and 2000, were classified as "oral laceration from accident while using device," says the report in the *American Journal of Preventive Medicine* (September 2004).

Spectacles of Death

Still more indoor perils, this time for shortsighted people: wearing metal-framed glasses could put you at risk of night blindness or even eye cancer, warns Pat Thomas, the American author of the 2003 book, *Living Dangerously: Are Everyday Toxins Making You Sick?* She claims that metal eyeglass frames can act as focusing antennae for electromagnetic forces from computers, electric toothbrushes, microwave ovens, power points, vacuum cleaners, and toasters—in fact, pretty much anything with a plug on it.

Killer Candles

Thomas is not the most relaxing person to have around the home: she also warns that candles can create clouds of dangerous chemicals. She quotes researchers in the *Journal of the American Medical Association* (2000, 284; 2:180) who bought candles from twelve different stores and found that a third had metallic wicks—and one tenth of these contained lead. The metal is still used by some candlemakers to stiffen candlewicks. "Every time you burn one of these lead-containing candles, you release significant amounts of neurotoxic lead into the atmosphere," Thomas says.

A further study in *Scientific Total Environment* (2002, 296; 1–3:159) warns that burning more than one candle in a room can push airborne-lead levels above U.S. safety limits. There goes that romantic dinner.

Indoor Sclerosis

If all that weren't enough to get you out of the house then consider this: staying indoors could help to end your life. We all know the manifold warnings about going out in the sun and getting skin cancer, but Australian researchers based at the University of Tasmania claim that the more sun you had as a child, the lower your chances of developing multiple sclerosis (MS).

They compared 136 people with MS with 272 randomly drawn people of similar ages, and found that those who had been out in the sun more than two to three hours a day between the ages of six and fifteen had a significantly lower risk of MS. Higher exposure in winter seemed more important than higher exposure in summer. They concluded in the *British Medical Journal* (2003, 327; 7410:316) that insufficient ultraviolet light may influence the development of the potentially fatal progressive disease.

Shade Lover's Carcinoma

Avoiding the sun can also make you more vulnerable to a range of common lethal cancers, claims Professor Cedric Garland of the University of California.

He recommends that you try to get some sun every day to allow adequate buildup of vitamin D, which reduces the risk of colon, breast, prostate, and other cancers. Professor Garland says in the *British Medical Journal* (2003, 327; 7425:1228), "Advice to avoid the sun would not be the best strategy for reducing overall incidence of cancer."

He advises, for example, that residents of northerly latitudes such as New York should aim for ten to fifteen minutes a day in the sun in the winter months when the weather allows, without sunscreen, to allow adequate synthesis of vitamin D.

How will you die?

Helpful safety experts have calculated your precise risk of getting killed in a whole range of mishaps. If you fear drowning in the bath, then you should be just as scared of suffocating in bed—the odds are exactly the same. Likewise, a venomous spider bite is as likely to bring about your demise as a fireworks accident.

Your odds for meeting the Grim Reaper via:

Complications of hospital care:	1 in 1,170
Riding a motorcycle:	1 in 1,295
Fatal air accident:	1 in 4,608
Being accidentally shot:	1 in 4,613
Tripping on level ground:	1 in 6,336
Falling off a ladder:	1 in 8,689
Choking on your own vomit:	1 in 9,372
Driving in a heavy truck:	1 in 9,702
Drowning in the bath:	1 in 10,948
Suffocating in bed:	1 in 10,948
Scalding by hot tapwater:	1 in 65,092
Hornet, wasp, or bee stings:	1 in 66,297
In a three-wheeled vehicle:	1 in 155,654
On foot:	1 in 610

Fireworks:	1 in 716,010
Venomous spiders:	1 in 716,010

Source: American National Safety Council's Lifetime Risk of Death Study, 2000.

On the Other Hand . . .

Rail journey is less risky than asteroid collision (but only just).

If the American scale were not precise enough, science has created another system to help us mortals fixate on our inevitable demise. Frank Duckworth, the eminent statistician and editor of the *Royal Statistical Society News*, has used figures from the *British Medical Journal* and the UK Health and Safety Executive to create the "Riskometer" to measure the risks of everyday living.

Like the Richter scale for earthquakes and the Beaufort scale for wind, the Duckworth Riskometer is a logarithmic scale. This means that things get much, much more dangerous the higher up you go in the risk rankings. Zero indicates simply living on the earth for one year; slightly more risky is taking a 160-kilometer train journey, rated at 0.3; at 8.0 is playing a game of Russian Roulette with a full chamber.

RISKOMETER RATINGS

8.0   Suicide; Russian roulette (with six bullets); jumping off Eiffel Tower; lying in front of an express train

7.2   Russian roulette (one round)

7.1	Continuing to smoke cigarettes (male age 35, 40 a day)
6.9	Continuing to smoke cigarettes (male age 35, 20 a day)
6.7	Continuing to smoke cigarettes (male age 35, 10 a day)
6.4	Deep-sea fishing (40-year career)
6.3	Rock climbing (over 20 years)
5.5	Accidental falls (newborn male)
5.5	Lifetime car travel (newborn male); dying while vacuuming, washing the dishes, or walking down the street
4.6	Murder (newborn male over whole lifetime)
4.2	Rock climbing (one session)
1.9	100-mile car journey (sober middle-aged driver)
1.7	1,000-mile flight
1.6	Asteroid impact in the lifetime of a newborn male
0.3	100-mile rail journey

Why are vacuuming the carpet and washing the dishes more risky than rock climbing? It's about the relative amount of time you spend doing them, says Duckworth: "I guess the risk of death in a lifetime of carrying out household chores would be between four and five on the scale."

Phone-Strike Fatalities

When seventeen-year-old New York student Jason Findley was found lying on a bed with a telephone receiver by his side, investigators were initially baffled—until they worked out that he had been electrocuted when lightning blasted an electrical surge through the telephone wire into his left ear and caused his heart to stop, reports the *New York Times* (February 16, 1986).

Phone-conducted lightning is not particularly rare. Officials of New Jersey Bell Telephone Company say telephone-related strikes are not uncommon, but fatal accidents are unusual. Several weeks before Findley's death, a New Jersey man was found unconscious with the phone in his hand after having received an electrical jolt. He survived.

In 2001, the *Journal of Laryngology & Otology* (2001, 115; 1:4) reported eighteen cases of ear injuries caused by lightning at the University Hospital of Split, Croatia, between 1984 and 1999. Not surprisingly, all were admitted complaining of "severe pain, tinnitus [ringing in the ears] and hearing impairment." Twelve of them suffered ruptured ear drums, though all were treated successfully. "Lightning survivors require additional psychotherapeutic treatment," the doctors recommend.

Dr. Christopher Andrews of Queensland, Australia, agrees about the need for therapy. He says about eighty people a year in Australia receive shocks from lightning surges while using telephones, and adds in the *Medical Journal of Australia* (1993, 157; 11–12:823) that victims do not only need care for shock and burns. They may require treatment with antidepressants, as there is a strong element of "no one else seems to understand" involved. Phone-strike survivors don't get much sympathy—their friends tend to fall down laughing.

HYPOCHONDRIA CAN KILL

Like you didn't have enough to fret about

If you are worried sick about your health, then you may be right to fret—you could fall victim to the *nocebo effect.* It is the placebo effect's evil dark-side brother. A placebo makes you get better because it helps you believe you will get better. The nocebo effect makes people who worry about illness become ill. And thus, paradoxically, it proves that hypochondria really isn't all in the mind.

Doctors have known about the placebo effect for thousands of years. Convince a person that some substance will make them recover from illness, and there is a strong chance it will do the trick—even if medically it doesn't actually work. Nowadays, the placebo pill used in medical drug trials—normally just a taste-free sugar tablet—can help to cure anything in up to 40 percent of the people who take it, by liberating the power of their self-belief. This can prove rather embarrassing if the expensive new wonder drug being tested against it doesn't do any better.

For many years, doctors have debated whether to work on "harnessing the placebo effect," but time after time they have backed off because it makes their scientific professional credibility look like witch-doctor voodoo. Placebo is all about harnessing the power of the mind, something that can't be measured, packaged, and sold—not least because it's so hit-and-miss. And doctors don't do voodoo, at least not officially.

The medical profession speaks even less of the nocebo effect—probably because it is so spooky—and also because it gives hypochondriacs something real to complain about. In one example of nocebo, researchers discovered that women who believe they are prone to heart disease are nearly four times as likely to die from it as women with similar risk factors who don't hold such fatalistic views.

The study, reported in the *Journal of the American Medical Association* (1996, 275; 5:345), covered more than five thousand women in Framingham, Massachusetts, a town whose population has been studied since 1948 in a long-term examination of three generations of Americans. The study results reinforced medics' understanding of the nocebo phenomenon, which was first identified more than four decades ago.

Nocebo (from the Latin "I will harm") seems a cruel testimony to the power of human imagination. "People are convinced that something is going to go wrong, and it is a self-fulfilling prophecy," says Arthur J. Barsky, a psychiatrist at Boston's Brigham and Women's Hospital. He warns in the *Journal of the American Medical Association* (2002, 287; 5:622) that doctors must pay closer attention to the nocebo effect. "From a clinical point of view, this is by no means peripheral or irrelevant," he says.

Barsky's roundup of previous studies shows how sixteen years ago, researchers at three medical centers undertook a study of aspirin and another blood thinner in heart patients and discovered that simply warning the aspirin-takers about possible side effects increased the number of patients who suffered them.

At two of the medical centers, patients were told of possible stomach problems, one of the most common side effects of repeated use of aspirin. At the other location, patients received no warning. The patients warned about the gastrointestinal trouble were almost three times as likely to suffer from it.

Another study, in the July 1981 *Pavlovian Journal of Biological Sciences,* reports how more than two thirds of a random sample of thirty-four college students reported mild headaches when told that a nonexistent electric current was passing through their heads.

Barsky has profiled the type of patient who is most likely to experience the nocebo effect of worse side effects and poorer results on a given drug. When he sees a patient with a history of vague, difficult-to-diagnose complaints who is sure that whatever therapy is prescribed will do little to battle the problem, he says, those low expectations are inevitably met. The treatments usually fail.

Court-Case Cripples

The nocebo effect also blights victims of accidents who become embroiled in long-running legal cases in pursuit of damages. This subset of the nocebo world has its own title, *compensation neurosis.* Sadly, the process of going through the courts means they never get better— especially if they win their case.

"Results of medical treatment are notoriously poor in patients with pending litigation after personal injury or disability claims," says a report in *Clinical Orthopedics* (1997; 336:94). These people are not malingering, it stresses. It is just that all the courtroom drama convinces their subconscious brains to ensure they stay wounded.

"Adversarial administrative and legal systems challenging the claimant to prove repeatedly that they are permanently ill
harden the conviction of illness," the
American report explains.

Worse still, even winning a fat compensation award at
the end of the case does not help: "Because any improvement in the claimant's health condition may result in denial of disability status in the future, the complainant is
compelled to guard against getting well and is left with
no honorable way to recover from illness."

Cultural Crashes

All this could well explain why, if you want to avoid
whiplash injury, you should not crash your car in North
America. Have the same neck-spraining accident in
Greece instead. The Greeks don't have a culture of making insurance claims for whiplash after car crashes—and
neither do they suffer any of the common whiplash
claimants' long-term disabling symptoms, say reports
from Alberta University, Canada.

The researchers wanted to discover why whiplash injuries are endemic in Canada but almost unknown in
Greece. They asked Canadians and Greeks to imagine
what injuries they would get from a neck-twisting motor
wreck. Half the Canadians said they might suffer long-
term disability, but almost none of the Greeks did, says
the report in the *Medical Science Monitor* (2003;
3:CR120-4).

What is behind the huge difference in expectations? It
is the chance of winning a big compensation payout in
litigious Western countries, says another Alberta Univer-

sity report, in *Orthopade* (2001, 30; 8:551). "In countries where whiplash syndrome does not exist, accident victims do not routinely hear reports of how it can cause severe long-term disability, so don't expect it can happen to them," the researchers say.

"They do not engage in a process that encourages hypervigilance for symptoms. They also do not engage in a process that engineers anxiety, frustration, and resentment from battling with insurance companies and proving that their pain is real. They will not amplify daily life's aches and pains. They will not attribute all these different sources of symptoms to chronic damage they believe the accident caused."

LOVE AND SEX

Is that Cupid's arrow, or has the Grim Reaper taken up archery?

Mistress Distress

Illicit relationships can kill you. Professor Graham Jackson, a consultant at St. Thomas's Hospital in London, England, claims that three quarters of sudden deaths during sex happen to people who are having affairs. This is particularly true of older people, says Jackson.

British statistics show that 1 percent of sudden deaths occur during sex, but you can boost your chances of a fatality by having intercourse with young and illicit partners. Jackson told a conference of the European Society for Sexual and Impotence Research in Hamburg (December 2002) that older, married men having flings with young mistresses are particularly at risk.

If that were not potentially embarrassing enough, a study of thirty-seven sex-related fatalities between 1972 and 1992, reported in Germany's *Zeitschrift für Kardiologie* (1999, 88; 1:44), found the majority had died of a heart attack, and "in most cases sudden death occurred during the sexual act with a prostitute."

The phenomenon of illicit sex-related deaths may be explained by clinical studies that claim to demonstrate that adultery works your heart harder than marital inter-course, which in turn is more stressful than masturba-tion.

The U.K. "sexologist" Dr. Alan Riley claims that heart rate increases by around 30 percent during intercourse, and by a maximum of 120 percent during orgasm. Mas-turbation, meanwhile, increases heart rate by around 29 percent, reaching a maximum increase of only 57 percent at orgasm.

In a 1983 study he reports how a forty-four-year-old man who had sex with both his wife and his mistress in the same day found that his heart recorded 92 beats per minute making love to his wife, and a high of 150 beats per minute with his mistress. He was supposed to be re-cuperating from a heart attack at the time.

Philanderers seeking to evade this cardiac curse might try asking their partners to go on top. But, according to Dr. Riley, position makes very little difference to the rate of cardiac exertion. Either way, men should expect on av-erage to expend a similar level of energy to that used when playing golf while carrying the clubs.

SEXY WIFE SHOCK

Ditch that attractive partner. Men with ugly wives live up to twelve years longer because they are not worried about them being unfaithful, Yale University scientists claimed in 1999 after studying the survival rates of sev-eral hundred couples.

Yale psychologist Edgar Dablen says in *The Globe and Mail* (April 2, 1999), "Men with attractive women are permanently jealous. They are always seeing competi-tion, which is an unhealthy and stressful situation."

Dangers of Dissent

Men, it seems, are immune to nagging—but their wives' lives could be in peril from frequent disagreements. Psychologists at Ohio State University studied thirty-one couples who were married for an·average of forty-two years, and found that wives' stress-hormone levels rose significantly at times when marital strife had been increased by partners' criticizing, interrupting, and disapproving.

The study, by Janice Kiecolt-Glaser and colleagues in *Psychosomatic Medicine* (1997; 59:339), found that the men's stress-hormone levels appeared unchanged. Perhaps they weren't listening.

Maybe if you are a man, the damage is primarily physical rather than emotional. A study by emergency-room doctors in Sunderland, England, found a significant number of men had punched their hands through windows following arguments with their partners. Seventy percent of them did it between the hours of 11 PM and 4 AM. More than half had to be hospitalized.

Inflatable Woman Warning

A new trend for giving women blow jobs may well reflect true sexual equality, but it also seems responsible for increasing numbers of women suffering mysterious chest pains, warn V. R. Jacobs and colleagues in the *Journal of the Society of Laporoendoscopic Surgeons* (2000, 4; 4:297).

They focus on the case of an otherwise young and healthy woman who arrived at the emergency department of Stanford University, California, complaining of recur-

rent chest pains. When x-rayed, she was found
to have air under her diaphragm, a spot where
air shouldn't be. The condition is called
pneumoperitoneum and is usually caused by
a perforated bowel or by surgeons accidentally
letting air into the body during an operation.

But both those causes were quickly ruled out. The
medics, in true baffled-doctor mode, resorted to asking
the woman about her lovemaking habits. She finally admitted to a liking for *vaginal insufflation*—having her
boyfriend blow up her for all he was worth.

This is a rather perilous form of blow job, though.
"Patients are often unaware of the open access between
the vagina and the abdomen," says Jacobs. "Vaginal insufflation can dilate genital organs and push remarkable
amounts of air into the abdomen. It can take several days
for the body to absorb the air, and the patient often does
not connect the pain with its cause."

You don't necessarily need a man to do it, either.
French pathologists report the tragic case of a woman
who killed herself by vaginal insufflation while masturbating. Their report, in the *International Journal of Legal
Medicine* (1990, 104; 1:59) says the forty-year-old woman
was using a carrot as a dildo when, bicycle-pump-style,
she managed to push enough air into herself to introduce
a lethal embolism—a bubble of gas—into her bloodstream.

The pathologists, based in Garches, say the case appears unprecedented, but speculate that this might be
due to the fact that investigators do not look for it as a
cause of death. They say it may also be that victims' partners deny that any dangerous behavior was going on—
and have also removed the carrot.

Leg-crosser's Impotence

Look out men, you risk infertility if you don't keep your knees apart. Professor Marc Goldstein says leg-crossing can lower a man's sperm production.

The professor of urology and director of the Center for Male Reproductive Medicine in New York says that sitting with one leg flung over the other for twenty minutes raises the temperature of the testes from around 32ºC, the optimum temperature for sperm-making, to between 36ºC and 37ºC. That could, he says, lower a man's fertility, though it won't show for eleven weeks, the Center points out, because it reportedly takes the body seventy-seven days to create sperm.

"Temperature is a very important factor in testicular function, and 2,000 years ago the Japanese used hot baths as a form of contraception. Anything above the optimum temperature could be detrimental," Professor Goldstein argues in the *Independent* newspaper (August 4, 1999).

Wet Nightmares

Talk in your sleep? Walk in your sleep? Drive in your sleep? You could be in danger of developing *sexsomnia,* or sleep-sex, according to Colin Shapiro, the director of Toronto University's Sleep and Alertness Clinic.

He cites eleven cases of people who unwittingly performed sex acts while asleep, often with unfortunate results. They did everything from normal intercourse to downloading porn from the Internet, he writes in the *Canadian Journal of Psychiatry* (2003, 48; 5:311). The patients had been referred to the clinic for other reasons and only mentioned the problem when questioned. "For many patients, embarrassment or a sense of guilt delayed medical enquiries," he says. "We anticipate that the number of potential cases is large, but sexual behavior in sleep is not recognized by physicians and hence is not considered worthy of history-taking or meriting referral for clinical examination."

Shapiro's cases include J.K., a married nightclub bouncer. He was referred to Shapiro after complaints by his wife, who claimed he frequently sexually assaulted her while sleeping. Criminal charges had been laid, and she was considering leaving him. He acknowledged attempting cunnilingus and intercourse while he was sleeping, but said he only knew of it because his wife had told him about it afterward. Our somnambulant sex-machine also had issues with snoring. When he was given an oxygen-feed device to stop his snoring, the sexual assaults stopped. But once he stopped wearing it two months later, the sexual assaults began again.

D.W., a forty-three-year-old divorced police officer, had previously been arrested and charged with drunk driving, but was acquitted on a defense of parasomnia (the medical term for general slumber-related weirdness). He was a frequent sleepwalker and sleep talker, and had started going for a drive while snoozing.

Sleep driving was not the only problem, though. He had a tendency to engage in intercourse when asleep. His two current girlfriends confirmed this habit. Shapiro's report says, "One describes him as 'a different person' during those activities—apparently he is a more amorous and gentle lover and more oriented toward satisfying his partner when he is asleep."

K.B., another police officer with a history of sleep driving (what is it with police officers?) was reported by his wife to have sleep-sex about once a month. "His wife describes him as more aggressive and more amorous at these times than when he is awake," the researchers report. "She says that at these times, 'There is no stopping him.' However, on one occasion when he grabbed her around the neck she slapped him hard and he immediately awoke and stopped the behavior."

In a third example cited by the researchers, a sixteen-year-old male sleepwalked into his uncle and aunt's bed and began fondling his uncle's testicles. In addition, his mother reports that she had found him downloading porn from the Internet in his sleep.

Some of us may feel particularly skeptical about this last case.

ONES TO AVOID

Sarah, Emma, Kelly, Louise, Claire, Lisa, Rachel, Clare, Michelle, Nicola

Young women who are prone to risky unprotected sex are more likely to be called Sarah, Emma, Kelly, or Louise than any other name. This is the claim of clinic doctors at a hospital in southern England who compiled the list, above, after studying the attendance records of nearly fifteen hundred women from ages sixteen to twenty-four to find out which names cropped up most.

They compared the findings with data from the Office of Population and Censuses indicating the most popular names over the last twenty years. Sharon and Tracey—the two names most associated in British popular culture with promiscuous young women, i.e. trailer trash—were far down the list of women's names most frequently seen as outpatients between April 1998 and March 1999 at the genito-urinary clinic of the Royal South Hants Hospital in Southampton, Hampshire.

Sharon entered the list way down at number thirty while Tracey was at thirty-five. Suspiciously enough, the two names were seen half as often as could have been expected, given their overall popularity. The doctors did concede, however, that some Sharons and Traceys might have visited the clinic under pseudonyms.

Amphibian of Love

Beware that French food, it could make your penis fall off, warn American university researchers. They seem to have solved a century-old medical mystery linking the consumption of frogs' legs to cases of *priapism*—painful and prolonged penile erection that might appear hilariously embarrassing, but can be seriously bad news—it can make the penis turn black and die.

The research is the first strong evidence that frogs' legs were behind two outbreaks of priapism among French soldiers in North Africa in 1861 and 1893. French doctors describe cases of "*erections douloureuses et prolongées*" among soldiers who had recently eaten frogs' legs. Precisely how long the troops were left standing at attention is unclear.

The doctors say the symptoms resembled those seen in men who had overindulged in a drug called cantharidin—popularly known as Spanish fly—which is extracted from a beetle for its supposed aphrodisiac qualities. In one of the North African cases, physicians dissecting a local frog found its guts full of these beetles. Until this study, however, nobody had shown that frogs eating the beetles could accumulate large enough concentrations of cantharidin to cause symptoms in humans who eat the frogs.

Thomas Eisner of Cornell University has now detected such concentrations in the legs of frogs fed cantharidin-producing beetles. The research report in *Chemoecology* says that a meal of the cantharidin-contaminated meat could contain more than enough of the compound to cause priapism. Gorging on these legs may lead to even more serious problems. People consuming two hundred to four hundred grams of Spanish fly–laden frog thighs in one meal could even risk death from cantharidin poisoning, he says.

Further Warning to Womanizers

Testicles can be the death of you, according to a study of eunuchs published in 1969, which showed that their life span was on average more than thirteen years longer than that of other males. Why? The geneticist David Gems, of University College, London, has an explanation: if you are an intact man, you wear yourself out chasing women.

In 1997 Gems found that a male nematode worm could live for twenty days when left on its own, but when males were kept together their lifespan fell to ten days. He says this is due to the stress of continual competition for territory and mates. Just to make sure, he tested male worms with genetic mutations that made them less active, reports *New Scientist* (May 24, 1997). They lived longest—thirty days.

Male marsupial mice live for years if they are castrated, instead of just a few sex-mad weeks when left intact.

"They spend five to eleven hours a day copulating," he says. Among humans, it is women who live longer, but men have the genetic potential to do better if they keep themselves to themselves, he argues.

Promiscuous Prostates

Men with interesting sex lives run a greater risk of contracting prostate cancer. A Swedish study says that while cigarettes and alcohol consumption may have little direct effect on the cancer, which kills nearly thirty thousand American men every year, frequent sex makes contracting the cancer more likely.

The report, in *Cancer Epidemiology Biomarkers Preview* (1996, 5; 7:509), says that men who lost their virginity earlier and had more sexual partners seem to have a higher incidence of prostate trouble. But cancer specialist Swen-Olof Andersson of Orebro Hospital is not prescribing therapeutic celibacy. "We don't think it's the sexual activity in itself, it might be some type of hormonal factor that also affects sexual drive," he says.

Breaking Condom News

Ooops: condom-wearing does not necessarily mean safe sex. Half the men who wear condoms have had a rubber break on them during intercourse, though their partners may very well not know, say researchers, backed by the Society for the Scientific Study of Sexuality, who questioned ninety-eight male students.

A third of the men who had experienced that worrisome moment of suddenly increased sensitivity hadn't told their partners. Why not? Nearly half admitted it was because they were about to orgasm. A third said they wanted to avoid responsibility for the break. The rest thought it best not to make their partner fret. The men who didn't tell were more likely to have slept around beforehand and to have ridden bareback when they did it, says the report in the *Journal of the American Medical Association* (1997, 278; 4:291).

Safe Socks Message

Then there's always the danger of a condom falling off inside a woman mid-sex. Australian scientists who studied prostitutes and "amateur" condom users have discovered that this is most likely to happen if you are a young, circumcised man, and put condoms on using the conventional, manufacturer-recommended method of rolling them down the penis.

The sex researchers fail to explain why circumcision might be a factor, but they strongly recommend, in the 1984 *Reproductive Health Matters* journal, that condom-wearers pull their prophylactics up like a sock. While there is a danger of sticking your fingers through the sides, they say the pull method is much easier than rolling, and therefore more effective—even if it does make you look odd.

Condom-donning success can mean little to safe sex, though, the scientists found. Half of the four hundred male interviewees subscribed to the "It's the thought that counts" school of sheath-wearing. They admitted that on at least one occasion, they had taken off a condom mid-sex and finished without it. That's hardly going to fool the viruses.

Ribbed for Sensitivity

Indian doctors have discovered another potential danger from prophylactics. You could suffocate on one.

Specialists at the Jaswant Rai Speciality Hospital in Meerut spent weeks giving a twenty-seven-year-old woman a range of antibiotics and tuberculosis drugs, but to no avail. Her persistent cough and fever, which had lasted six months, would not go away.

So they x-rayed her chest and found that one lung had partially collapsed around a mystery object. A video probe was popped in there, revealing an "inverted bag-like structure." It was removed with forceps and turned out to be an old condom.

"Detailed retrospective history confirmed accidental inhalation of the condom during fellatio," report the doctors in the *Indian Journal of Chest Disease and Allied Science* (2004, 46; 1:55).

INFECTION? WHAT INFECTION?

How well would you trust a foreign lover? The following figures allegedly show the likelihood of people from different nationalities admitting to their partners that they have got something nasty down there (*Durex Global Survey*, December 2003):

Austria	83 percent
United Kingdom	80 percent
Australia	80 percent
France	72 percent

Czech Republic	55 percent
Vietnam	44 percent
Singapore	39 percent
Thailand	20 percent
Taiwan	13 percent
Malaysia	10 percent

Note, however, that this survey asked people whether they *would* tell their partners if they *did* have a disease. So the survey might just prove that Malaysians told the interviewers the truth, while many Austrians are barefaced liars.

Masturbation Mayhem

Go easy with those one-handed fantasies: autoerotic asphyxiation is not an uncommon form of death. And from Germany comes a salutary caution about the use of army-surplus gear in self-sex.

Researchers writing in the *Arkiv für Kriminologie* (1997, 200; 3–4:65) tell of a nineteen-year-old man who purchased an ex–air force G suit for the purposes of solitary pleasure. This is a pressure-suit worn by jet fighter pilots that applies pneumatic tourniquets to parts of the body in tight high-speed turns, and thus stops blood from rushing to the pilot's head or feet, preventing blackouts.

Things took a strange turn with our young onanist, however. He inflated the suit with a twelve-volt air compressor, covered his head with three masks and a motorcycle helmet, and managed to tie up his arms and legs. The cause of death was a massive compression of the thorax.

Fatal Traction

Meanwhile, men who dig masochistic masturbation are in peril of suffering lethal tractor fetishes, warn forensic scientists at Ventura County, California. They report two cases in which men used the hydraulic shovels on tractors to "suspend themselves for masochistic stimulation."

"One man developed a romantic attachment to a tractor, even giving it a name and writing poetry in its honor," says the report in the *Journal of Forensic Sciences* (1994, 39; 5:1143). He died accidentally while asphyxiating himself for pleasure by hanging himself from the machine by his neck. The forensic officers say that literature he left behind suggests he enjoyed the sense of being strangled.

The other man in the report became pinned to the ground under a shovel after suspending himself from it by the ankles.

Terrible Turn-ons

For another autoerotic death shock turn to the *American Journal of Forensic Medical Pathology* (2003, 24; 1:92), where J. C. Schott and colleagues tell of an eighteen-year-old man wearing two brassieres who was found dead in his bedroom by his brother. Two wet green cloths were under the brassiere cups connected to the electric mains via two metal washers and an electrical cord.

"Literature depicting nude women was found near the victim," write the forensic officers from Kentucky University. An autopsy revealed second- and third-degree burns of the mammary regions. Death was attributed to accidental self-electrocution.

And medicolegal doctors at Graz University, Austria, report how a man died of electrocution after attaching one electrode to his anus and then accidentally touching the other electrode against his chest while he was attempting to connect it to his penis. The shock caused his heart to fail. The poor man's parents tried to hide both the cable and pornographic magazines to conceal the cause of death, but failed to fool the doctors, says the report in the *American Journal of Forensic Medical Pathology* (1998, 19; 2:190).

Milk-Bottle Bother

How can you while away seventeen hours with your penis trapped in a milk bottle? Ask the Japanese victim of penile incarceration, reported in the journal *Hinyokika Kiyo* (1988, 34; 3:514). The thirty-eight-year-old man arrived at Osaka City University Medical School after he had trapped his penis in a milk bottle all the previous evening.

Once the patient had summoned up the courage to go to the hospital—or decided he really needed to use the bathroom—the bottle "was successfully removed by means of a glass cutter and hammer without any complication," report the doctors.

There must be something particularly alluring about Japanese milk bottles. The doctors say they know of another fifty-six of their countrymen who have trapped their penises in exactly the same way.

Murder wrap

Getting trapped and wrapped was the awful fate of a male autoeroticist reported in the *American Journal of Forensic Medical Pathology* (1985, 6; 2:151). It tells of how the victim died as a result of "jeopardizing himself" by tightly wrapping his body in plastic wrap, with an airway out of his cocoon in the form of a snorkel tube. He was busily engaged in masturbation when he apparently lost his mouthpiece. He attempted to use a knife to cut himself out, but failed and was found suffocated.

VISE SCREAM

For something still rarer, weirder, and far more German, we return to the *Arkiv für Kriminologie* (2001, 207; 5–6:148) and a report from Berlin's Humboldt University, titled "An unusual autoerotic accident: sexual pleasure from peritoneal pain."

It reports the unfortunate story of a twenty-three-year-old man who got his sexual thrills by jabbing his abdomen with sharp instruments. For this purpose he clamped two knife blades into a vise suspended from a rope-pulley so that he could lower it onto himself to pierce his skin with the knife tips.

Unfortunately, one of the ropes broke and the vise with the knives fell onto the man's belly, piercing a major artery, and he bled to death. This, to the authors' knowledge, has been the first-ever report of a fatal autoerotic accident in which sexual pleasure was to be obtained from painful irritation of the peritoneum.

Overdressed for Sex

Such sexual shenanigans are not only popular with Germans and Japanese people; Australians also feature strongly in the annals of single-handed death. The Forensic Science Centre in Adelaide, South Australia, reports a series of masturbation-related fatalities in the *American Journal of Forensic Medical Pathology* (2000, 21; 1:65).

Saddest was the case of a forty-six-year-old man found dead in the bushland clothed in a dress, female undergarments, and seven pairs of stockings and panty hose. The underwear had been cut to enable him to access his genitals. Unfortunately, it was high summer, 39°C— time for a light shirt and shorts, not layers of women's clothing.

The victim was declared dead through hyperthermia— massive overheating of the body, due to a combination of excessive clothing and high ambient temperature, says the report.

Limb Love

If you would give your right arm to have a powerful orgasm, you may have developed *apotemnophilia,* a fetish shared by only about two hundred people around the world in which sexual gratification is derived from the removal of a limb.

It's not just bad for the patients. In 1999, an unlicensed physician who amputated a healthy leg for $15,000 to satisfy his elderly patient's apotemnophilia was sentenced to fifteen years in prison after the botched operation killed the man. John Ronald Brown, seventy-seven, had been a doctor for almost thirty years until his medical license was withdrawn in 1977 for negligence.

Brown chopped off the left leg of Philip Bondy, a seventy-nine-year-old New York apotemnophiliac, in a crude operation in Mexico, and buried the severed limb to hide the evidence. Bondy was left to recuperate in a hotel room, and died two days later of gangrene poisoning.

How Did That Get Up There?

Be wary of leaving tubular objects sitting upright on the shower stall floor. "Slipping over and falling backward onto [insert name of offending object here]" appears to be the primary cause of mortally embarrassed people getting things jammed up their rectums and needing doctors to remove them.

What are the most frequently misplaced objects? Doctors David Busch and James Starling of Wisconsin report the top ten items in *Surgery* (1986, 100; 3:512) after discovering 182 cases written up in the world's medical journals.

OBJECT	NUMBER REMOVED
Glass or ceramic bottle or jar	32
Vibrator	23
Dildo	15
Glass or cup	12

Stick or broom handle	10
Lightbulb	7
Tube	6
Carrot	4
Cucumber	3
Cattle horn	3

Mortifying shame can be the least of a victim's problems. Gordian Fulde, the emergency department director at St. Vincent's Hospital, Darlinghurst, Australia, says retrieving rectum-jammed objects is often far harder—and much more dangerous—than sticking them up there in the first place.

One German team managed to remove a firmly lodged apple only by mulching it with an argon laser, he says, while Athens doctors have resorted to using obstetric forceps to extract difficult objects. A rural Australian team used a suction plunger to pull out a glass bottle.

But one in ten cases still needs an operation, either to remove the object or to repair a perforated bowel. Such poor patients may end up with a colostomy, Fulde warns in the *Medical Journal of Australia* (1998; 169:670).

Fracture of the Penis

Steer clear of overenthusiastic sex if you are fortysomething. Around 1 out of every 175,000 hospital admissions is for a fractured penis. Ouch.

It is caused when the erect penis is forcibly bent—in most cases during sexual intercourse. Dr. Frederick Klein, the assistant professor of urology at the Medical College of Virginia in Richmond, explains: "The patient hears a 'crack' or 'pop,' and his penis immediately shrinks and then swells painfully and turns black and blue."

The penis usually bends to the side opposite the injury; if the left corpus cavernosum is ruptured, for example, the penis will be bent to the right. Dr. Klein and colleagues report in the *Journal of Trauma* (1985, 25; 11:1090) that patients are hospitalized for about two weeks on average, and good results are achieved in about 75 percent of cases treated with surgery.

A global survey in the *British Journal of Surgery* (2002, 89; 5:555) declares that penile fracture is "not rare." It found that 1,331 cases were reported in medical journals between January 1935 and July 2001. Most reports were from the Mediterranean region. Most patients were in their forties.

FORGETTABLE SEX

Japanese neuropsychiatrists at Tokushima University Medical School report how one of their female patients developed an alarming episode of complete amnesia after enjoying vigorous intercourse. Sudden isolated bouts of complete memory loss and confusion in otherwise healthy people are called *transient global amnesia.* Victims forget where they are and the identity of the people they are with (which is sometimes convenient).

The Tokushima scientists report how sex caused the woman's amnesiac condition in the *Japanese Journal of Psychiatry and Neurology* (1993, 47; 1:13). They speculate that it may be sparked by heightened blood pressure dropping rapidly after intercourse, causing a temporary fall in the brain's oxygen supply.

This might explain how the sufferers' ability to store new memories is also temporarily lost. The condition can also be caused by heavy exercise, particularly swimming in cold water. Attacks can last for several hours.

But in 1998, two blood specialists from America's Johns Hopkins University suggested in the *Lancet* (1998, 352; 9139:1557) that the problem may be caused by tensing the abdominal muscles and straining, the way women do when giving birth—or having sex. This, they say, may cause a rush of blood to the brain—and it could affect one person in every ten thousand.

Soccer-cup celibacy

Bad news for soccer wives. The healthcare market research company, Isis, claims that big sports events can ruin your love life.

It says a significant dip in prescriptions for erectile dysfunction drugs such as Viagra occurred during the soccer World Cup in the summer of 2002—a peak period for men sitting on the couch in front of the television with their pals and a few cold beers.

The World Cup weeks saw the only drop in U.K. prescriptions over a two-year period: from around twenty-five thousand a month, down to the thirteen thousand mark. Isis claims the two bouts of low-scoring are linked. Soccer? It's better than sex.

Large Bust or Bust

If you are a woman with small breasts, you are also likely to be underendowed in the intelligence department.

GP newspaper (December 15, 2003) reports how a study by the University of Chicago discovered that women with a breast size of D cup or greater score on average ten IQ points higher than those with an A or B cup.

But having impressive frontal lobes does not necessarily mean a ticket to academic success, say the statisticians. They suggest that well-built women are in fact viewed as less intelligent because men pay more attention to their cleavage than to their conversation. Talk to the face, guys.

HISTORY'S TOP HYPOCHONDRIACS

I told you I was ill . . .

Artistic, sensitive, ambitious? Many of the world's finest minds fall prey to illnesses cooked up by their fertile imaginations. Fortunately, hypochondria can plague evil megalomaniacs, too.

One of the classic ironies of hypochondria is that you can spend so many years crying wolf that no one else worries when something really does go wrong. Take the French playwright Molière, a notorious hypochondriac, who used his lifetime's experience of health gripes to create Argon, the central character of his play, *The Imaginary Invalid*. Argon, like Molière, was always complaining about illness and fearing he was but a step away from the grave. Molière played the theatrical part himself—and sadly did it only too well. He died in 1672, on the evening of the satire's fourth performance, after suffering a coughing fit and hemorrhage onstage. His fellow actors had dismissed his earlier protestations of illness, so he never got to see a doctor in time.

The American composer Leonard Bernstein met a similar fate. He spent fifteen years in thrall to a variety of imaginary ailments. So when he started complaining of headaches, then suffered a blackout onstage and complained of smelling burning rubber, the doctors who checked him out were skeptical and said, ho hum, nothing seems to be wrong. After four days of hospital tests, they concluded he was suffering from a nervous affliction, probably self-induced. His medical form decreed, "Most likely hysteria."

His psychoanalyst also concluded that Bernstein's symptoms were all in the mind. One neurologist suggested he undergo a spinal tap, just to be sure there were no problems with his brain. But it is a painful procedure, and Bernstein would not go through with it. Five months later, and to everyone's surprise but Bernstein's, the composer fell into a coma. Several hours of surgery were to no avail. He had been suffering from a brain tumor and died in October 1990.

Should you wish to argue that hypochondria is a disease of the overactive imagination, then there is no shortage of artists, writers, actors, thinkers, and megalomaniacs to support you. Bernstein's fellow composer, Igor Stravinsky, was not only a hypochondriacal danger to himself. His family got caught up in his ill-health enthusiasms, too. Stravinsky went to see a doctor in every city he visited, and was also constantly swallowing pills that he prescribed for himself. In 1934, soon after his son, Theodore, needed emergency surgery for a ruptured appendix, Stravinsky had his own healthy appendix removed "as a precaution." Cautious Igor ordered that the same operation be performed on his other three children, too.

Enrico Caruso was also the careful sort. The operatic tenor equipped himself with an armory of atomizers, gargling fluids, migraine medicines, and cold and cough cures wherever he traveled. He was also desperate to avoid catching skin complaints, so took his own linen with him to hotels. Before he occupied a suite, it had to be sprayed with disinfectant. He would bathe and change his clothes after walking in the street or being in close contact with strangers in a public place. Before going to bed, he saw that a mattress and piles of pillows were arranged around him on the floor in case he fell out of bed in his sleep and hurt himself.

At least he had not been exposed to medical training. The father of evolutionary theory, Charles Darwin, began a lifetime of hypochondriacal suffering as a medical student, where many young people learn to imagine the horrors of encroaching illness. The British Medical Association nowadays warns proto-medics of this peril, but Darwin, as an evolutionist, would be pleased to know he was one of the first examples. He was a big man but sensitive, too: "It seems, as soon as the stimulus of mental work stops, my whole strength gives way," he complained. Not only did he suffer from psychosomatic exhaustion, but Darwin also labored with chronic intestinal disorders that seemed more in his mind than in his gut.

Psychoanalysts have had a jolly time suggesting that his stomach problems were rooted in the guilt he felt about toppling thousands of years of religious beliefs. But it wasn't all gloom and doom. Darwin liked sex—he married twice and produced several illegitimate children—and he prescribed sexual intercourse as a cure for hypochondria. At least it took his mind off things. A later scientific revolutionary, Sigmund Freud, would have agreed with this diagnosis: his simple explanation for hypochondria was that it is the product of the victim's libidinal energies being directed at their own body (in plainer terms, the victim is screwing himself). It is not, Freud said, a matter for psychiatry.

But sex was a cause, rather than a cure, for the writer James Boswell's bodily obsessions. The eighteenth-century writer and biographer of Samuel Johnson was persistently haunted by the idea that he had contracted an incurable venereal disease. This may well have been sexual guilt. He had indeed caught a dose of VD as a youth, but the infection had cleared up. To distract himself from his syphilitic fixation, Boswell used to go out to watch public hangings.

And Boswell always needed cheering up. He sank into his most severe hypochondria in 1763 when he went to study law at Utrecht University in the Netherlands. "A deep melancholy seized upon me. I groaned with the idea of living all winter in so shocking a place," he complained in his journal. "I was worse and worse the next day. All the horrid ideas you can imagine recurred upon me . . . I sunk quite into despair. I thought at length the time was come that I should grow mad."

Boswell believed his affliction was hereditary. His mother, he said, was "an extremely delicate girl, very hypochondriac."

The poet Alfred Lord Tennyson, mean- while, was fixated with the dread possibility of his eyesight failing. He worried about blindness his entire life. Ordinary floaters across his field of vision worried him. He called them "animals," and wrote to his aunt, "These animals you mention are very distressing and mine increase weekly; in fact I almost look forward with certainty to being blind some of these days." Tennyson died in his eighties. His eyesight had remained tolerably good.

That is another of the great ironies of hypochondria— so many of its sufferers live to a ripe old age—and achieve far more than the vast majority of people who feel hap-

pily healthy. Immanuel Kant, the metaphysical philoso-
pher, wrote: "Between health and insanity lies hypochondria," and he was one to know.

The creator of the categorical imperative once claimed
that his headaches were due to a special kind of electricity in the cloud systems. He also suspected that his organs
were jammed together so tightly that they prevented him
from breathing properly. Despite his lifetime of hypochondria, he never met with a serious illness, and died
on February 12, 1804, at the age of seventy-nine.

Florence Nightingale had an even longer struggle
with her imagined illnesses on her way to lasting fame.
Biographers speculate that it was her traumatic battle
against death, disease, and medical politics during the
Crimean War that turned her into a sickness obsessive. In
1857, the year after she returned from Crimea, she took
to her bed, convinced that her life was in imminent
danger.

Meanwhile, she continued to follow her vocation, to
campaign for the establishment of nursing as a profession, and to set up London's Nightingale School for
Nurses. She also pioneered the use of statistics in medicine. Her biographer, Lytton Strachey, wrote, "She remained an invalid, but an invalid of curious character—an
invalid who was too weak to walk downstairs and who
worked harder than most cabinet ministers . . . her illness, whatever it may have been, was not inconvenient."
Like all hypochondriacs, she was proved right in the
end—though she had to wait until 1910, when she was
ninety years old, for death to catch up with her.

Another celebrity homebound achiever, Marcel Proust,
made a literary career from novels peopled with sickness
and morbid psychology. There can be few better examples of that ancient piece of literary advice: write about

what you know. "Infirmity alone makes us take notice and learn, and enables us to analyse processes which we would otherwise know nothing about," wrote Proust, and he certainly knew a lot about infirmity.

Proust had a "severely troubled" stomach and reportedly ate only once a day from a select group of foods. He experienced terrible insomnia at night and spent his life as a perpetual invalid, passing through a succession of colds and fevers. He stayed indoors as much as possible because he was terrified of germs—and even refused to open windows. He also thought that he was allergic to strong light, and said his skin was so sensitive, he could not use soap—so he avoided baths and preferred instead to dab himself with a collection of damp towels. Noise from neighbors drove him nearly mad—which is bad news if you stay in all day—hence his life in a cork-lined, sound-insulated room.

In his novel, *In Search of Lost Time*, Proust wrote, "For each illness that doctors cure with medicine, they provoke it in ten healthy people by inoculating them with the virus that is a thousand times more powerful than any microbe: the idea that one is ill." Fortunately for hypochondriac posterity, our Frenchman completed all seven volumes of *Remembrance of Things Past* before he contracted pneumonia and died at the age of fifty-one.

But you don't have to start out as an effetely nervous wreck to end up a hypochondriacal recluse. How about beginning as an oil tycoon, record-breaking daredevil pilot, political intriguer, movie mogul, and the man once nicknamed the "world's greatest womanizer"?

That would be Howard Hughes, who started his career as a millionaire playboy and ended it as an emaciated hermit. Things began to go wrong for Hughes when he was severely injured in a serious plane crash in 1946 and subsequently became addicted to morphine. Later he moved to Las Vegas and began increasingly to shun society as a severe hypochondriacal fear of infection took hold. During his eighteen years of seclusion he had a huge air purifier installed into a car that took up most of the trunk and cost more than the limousine itself.

Up in the hotel he owned, he had his food delivered in paper bags that had previously remained untouched in a sealed cupboard for two years. The drivers had to wear white cotton hospital gloves when they carried the bags. Hughes extracted the food—mostly Hershey bars and milk—with Kleenex wrapped around his hand.

He had strict rules over the delivery of magazines. Three copies of the same magazine were always presented to him. Hughes would reach out, his hands and arms swathed in paper, and delicately remove the middle magazine from its companions. He would repeat, over and over again, instructions for the other magazines to be burned. He also used a minimum of fifteen tissues to open his cabinets. His last political cause was to try to stop underground nuclear testing in Nevada, because he was so terrified of radiation.

Is capitalism in itself a cause of hypochondria? Not if you are Nicolae Ceaucescu. When the communist dictator of Romania visited a Transylvanian castle early in his rule, it was not the prospect of vampires that rattled him. His guide around Peles Castle, a fine German Renaissance building and one of Romania's national treasures, was rash enough to point out that some of the castle woodwork was afflicted by fungus.

The fungus was no danger to humans, but Ceaucescu had a morbid fear of infections, and left the place there and then, never to return. There was a bright side—Ceaucescu's paranoia meant he left the area well alone—

never subjecting it to the brutalist concrete moderniza-
tion that wrecked places such as Bucharest.

Ceaucescu was not the only megalomaniac to have
given hypochondriacs a bad name. He pales in comparison with Adolf Hitler, both in despotism and health
paranoia. In fact, Hitler has a strong claim to being
history's greatest hypochondriac. To begin with the mundane items, he constantly fretted about his health, was
fanatical about cleanliness, never drank alcohol, never
smoked, and never allowed anyone to smoke in his
presence.

When he learned that he had shaken hands with a former prostitute who was marrying one of his generals, he
immediately took multiple showers. His hyperambitious
deputy, Martin Bormann, managed to have one of Hitler's
closest friends, Heinrich Hoffmann, banned from Hitler's
company. Knowing about Hitler's hypochondria, Bormann scurrilously informed him that Hoffmann was carrying a contagious disease. A distressed Hitler refused to
have Hoffmann come anywhere near him.

There were other worries, too. Hitler's mother had
died of cancer and Adolf desperately feared he would
be stricken with the disease as well. His fear intensified
when he had surgery to remove a polyp from his throat.
Even though he was reassured by doctors that the
polyp was benign, he was convinced that it was cancer.
He wrote his last will and testament in 1938, certain that
he was going to die before he completed his political
plans.

Hitler became even more obsessed with his health after the failed assassination attempt on him in 1944. His
doctor prescribed drugs of his own design that contained
hemlock. Hitler gulped so many pills he was slowly poisoning himself. Tremors in his right hand became acute,

· and he rarely allowed photographs or film of him after July 1944.

But the dictator did not just keep his hypochondria to himself. He tried to instill it into an entire country. One of his party's slogans instructed the German people: "Your body belongs to the nation! Your body belongs to the Führer! You have the duty to be healthy! Food is not a private matter!"

Hitler's exhortations are reminiscent of the new brand of healthy-eating messages that Western governments increasingly use to imply that being overweight is not only unhealthy, but an irresponsible burden on the state's meager health and welfare resources. Body fascism? Health Nazism? Could it all be the product of power-crazed politicians' contagious hypochondria?

EAT, DRINK, AND . . .

Be merry, for tomorrow you may worry yourself dead

Misfortune Cookies

The trouble with Chinese food, the old saying goes, is that after you've had one meal, you get hungry after a half an hour and want another one. Not if you suffer from *Chinese restaurant syndrome.*

The symptoms, identified in 1968 by Dr. Robert Byck, a Yale Medical School psychiatrist and brain researcher, are headache, sweats and hot flushes, chest pain, numbness or burning in and around the mouth, and a sense of facial pressure or swelling. Medical tests show victims have abnormal heart rhythm, rapid heart rate, and restricted breathing.

Most people recover from mild cases of Chinese restaurant syndrome on their own. But some researchers claim it can be life-threatening, with all the symptoms of severe anaphylactic shock reaction, such as throat-swelling.

Why would an innocent sweet-and-sour dish wreak such havoc? The *New York Times* (August 21, 1999) reports that Byck blamed the flavor enhancer monosodium glutamate (MSG) for sparking reactions in susceptible people. He did his research in a restaurant near his lab, and his findings led to MSG being banned from American baby food. But the claims have sparked widely conflicting reports from research studies, with many arguing that the link is not proven.

Monosodium glutamate is chemically similar to one of the brain's neurotransmitters, glutamate, and the anti-MSG camp claims this is significant. The additive is also blamed for glutamate-induced asthma and, less obviously, *hot dog headache,* by chemotherapy experts at Mount Sinai Medical Center, New York, in *Medical Hypotheses* (1992, 38; 3:185). While the link remains unproved, food vendors will continue to pep up their dishes with MSG.

Hot dogs should carry a health warning anyway, according to John Peters, a University of Southern California epidemiologist, who claims in the journal *Cancer Causes and Control* (1994, 5; 2:195) that children who eat more than twelve hot dogs a month appear to have nine times the normal risk of developing childhood leukemia. As well as *hot dog–related leukemia,* the journal also reports that children born to fathers who ate many hot dogs before conception have a significantly increased risk of developing brain tumors.

Chicken Ouch Mein

Headaches and possible death are not the only threats you face when going for a Chinese meal. Using chopsticks may cause arthritis.

A study of more than twenty-five hundred residents of Beijing found that osteoarthritis is more common in hands that are used to operate chopsticks, specifically the thumb and the second and third joints on the first and third fingers, which are most stressed by chopstick use, researchers report in *Arthritis and Rheumatology* (2004, 50; 5:1495).

Dr. David Hunter of the Boston University School of Medicine and colleagues interviewed 2,507 sixty-year-old residents in randomly selected Beijing neighborhoods. "This study suggests that chopsticks may play a role in the development of hand osteoarthritis," Hunter says. "We recommend further biomechanical research to evaluate the forces involved in chopstick use."

Pain on a Stick

What could be more innocently pleasurable than a summertime ice cream? But beware *ice-cream headache,* which normally hits victims twenty-five to sixty seconds after the first bite, can be blindingly intense and may affect up to one in three people.

Dr. David Roby, a neurologist at America's Temple University Hospital, warns in a news release dated June 29, 2004, that the headaches are like miniature migraines, and particularly affect migraine sufferers. Although no one knows for sure how ice cream can trigger pain, "The general belief is that the sudden change in temperature causes an overstimulation of the central nervous system," says Roby. Summertime, unsurprisingly, is high season for the problem, he adds.

SAUSAGE SCARE

Eating blood sausage before undergoing a cancer screening could result in unnecessary hospital procedures.

Stomach surgeons gathered volunteers from the English town of Bury, known as the black-pudding capital of the world, and asked them to eat the local sausage delicacy, which is made from congealed pigs' blood.

The research team, from Frenchay Hospital, Bristol, United Kingdom, discovered that black pudding can produce false positive results in screening tests for cancers of the colon and rectum. The tests look for blood in people's stools, and can't tell the difference between pigs' blood and human blood, says the report in the *British Medical Journal* (2002, 325; 7378:1444).

The doctors then surveyed one hundred people about their eating habits and discovered some 63 percent of them occasionally succumb to the temptation of a sausage full of pig plasma. This led them to conclude that, thanks to black puddings, more than twice the expected number of people may test positive for colon and rectal cancer—and be sent for needless further investigations.

DRINKING FOR STONERS

Cutting your alcohol intake is in all probability a good thing. But sobriety could increase women's chances of developing gallstones. Females who like a drink or three are less likely to develop gallstone problems, say researchers from the Harvard School of Public Health. It is not only one's inhibitions that are soluble in alcohol: the booze seems to hinder the stones' formation.

The researchers studied more than eighty thousand nurses to discover the link, which they report in the *American Journal of Clinical Nutrition* (2003, 78; 2:339). And it doesn't matter what type of alcohol you drink.

The authors suggest, however, that "Despite the inverse association between regular, moderate alcohol intake and gallstone disease, interested patients should discuss the health effects of alcohol consumption with their healthcare providers, who can help determine the patients' overall health risks and benefits, as well as provide an individual clinical recommendation."

Better from the Bottle . . .

That bottle-sucking wino could be drinking more safely than you. Italian researchers say you can get dangerous amounts of lead in your bloodstream by drinking from shiny new lead crystal glasses. But it depends on what you drink out of them. Cola drinks are safe because they draw very little lead from the glass. But who drinks cola out of crystal?

White wine, which you are far more likely to drink from crystal glasses, draws the highest level of lead of any of the liquids studied, reports the journal *Food Additives and Contamination* (2000, 17; 3:205).

Once you start washing your glasses, however, the rules change. When a crystal glass has been through the dishwasher three times, the levels of lead in wine stay the same, but the levels of lead in the cola drinks increase as the surface of the glass becomes roughened and more likely to leech out lead, say researchers at the glass study institute, the Stazione Sperimentale del Vetro of Murano-Venezia, Italy.

Soft Tap Heart Attacks

Health promoters are forever at us to drink more water. But your domestic supply could be boosting your risk
of a heart attack, a study claims.

People who live in areas with soft tapwater have significantly increased risk of cardiac death compared with
their hard-water counterparts, say researchers in Finland.
They studied nineteen thousand men between ages
thirty-five and seventy-four who had suffered heart attacks, and found that for every unit increase in water
softness, there is a 1 percent increase in the risk of coronary failure.

The researchers claim in the *Journal of Epidemiology
and Community Health* (2004, 58; 2:136) that the findings explain why heart attack rates vary by up to 40 percent from region to region. They examined the minerals
dissolved in hard water, and suggest that its higher fluo-
ride levels may help protect your heart.

But not all hard water is good news. For every micro-
gram of dissolved iron per liter in some types of hard water, the heart-attack risk increases by an average of 4
percent, the epidemiologists say, and for every micro-
gram of copper per liter of water, it rises by 10 percent.

Cuppaholics Anonymous

Alcohol, as we all know, can drive you into the arms
of strangeness. But tea and coffee can have the same
effect—if you fall victim to *caffeinism.*

Some medical experts believe caffeinism is similar to

alcoholism in that sufferers are the last to realize they have a problem. Symptoms can include confusion, restlessness, nervousness, insomnia, sweating, and palpitations. In extreme cases, manic behavior and panic disorders can develop. In one recorded case, a British soldier serving in the Indian army was believed to have been blinded by drinking too much tea.

The condition last came to light in 1997 as part of the defense case of another British trooper, a senior army officer accused of false accounting. Major David Senior, a decorated helicopter pilot in the Army Air Corps, had drunk up to a gallon of tea every day for twenty years.

Charles Gabb, his defense counsel, said in Major Senior's court martial proceedings: "On first hearing this some people may laugh, but he was known as a teetotaller who drank an enormous quantity of tea." He announced that his client had not been dishonest in any way but may have made a genuine mistake with paperwork relating to the fund because of his condition.

The *Daily Mail* (June 13, 1997) reports that all the charges of false accounting and theft against him were dropped.

Legless Dope

Doctors at Heidelberg University's Chirurgische Klinik und Poliklinik reported an unusual case of acute compartmental syndrome, a serious condition in which blood flow becomes trapped in a part of the body, cutting off the oxygen that tissues need. It is more often seen in patients who have been crushed by falling buildings.

This victim however, was found several hours after he had smoked several cannabis joints and fallen soundly asleep in the lotus position, says the report in *Chirurg* (1997, 68; 8:829). The doctors say that by passing out in a cross-legged posture, he catastrophically blocked the flow of several major arteries. When they examined him, he was in severe pain and his legs were stiff and swollen. They had to cut into his legs to relieve the pressure, but the blood-flow crisis had already prompted his kidneys to fail.

Fortunately, after two weeks of dialysis, the patient's kidneys started working again, and eventually he made a full recovery.

Crash Diet? Witness the Scars

Obesity is currently touted as a massive health threat, but certain stringent diets run you the risk of harming your looks. The American Academy of Cosmetic Surgery issued the warning after discovering that vegetarians on poorly balanced food intakes often suffer scarring and delayed healing when they have relatively superficial operations.

The Academy says weight-conscious eaters are at significantly increased risk of scarring if they restrict their diets and cut out wound-healing nutrients. It says in the *Journal of the American Medical Association* (1995, 273; 12:910) that these include albumin, which is found in proteins; glucose from carbohydrates; essential fatty acids; vitamins A, C, K, and B-complex; and the minerals zinc, copper, iron, and manganese.

You might want to pork up before that tummy tuck.

SLIM HEALTH CHANCES

If you are slim, you may have no reason to scoff. Losing weight may not be the great health-enhancer anyway. It might not be fatness, but fitness, that counts, say doctors who warn that thin couch potatoes are more at risk of illness than fat people who exercise.

Unfit men who are not obese have almost three times the death rate of other men who are fit but medically obese, say researchers at the Cooper Institute for Aerobics Research in Dallas, Texas, which studied twenty-five thousand males for nearly twenty years.

The institute's director of research, Steven Blair, told a London conference in July 1997 that when researchers normally study obese people, they discover illnesses that they blame on fat. In fact, it is their laziness that's unhealthy, he claimed at the Health Education Authority conference.

Who Ordered the Hemorrhage?

Gourmet food—all those overpriced exotic dishes comprising bits of endangered species swimming in rich sauces—is as much a threat to your finances as it is to your arteries. But you could become obsessed with the stuff if you suffer a fairly common form of brain hemorrhage.

Researchers cite the case of a patient who suffered a

hemorrhage and became so obsessed with rich food that eating soon became the only topic of conversation that interested him. In his daily diary, he recorded yearnings for sausage with mashed potatoes covered in butter, and scallops of duck smothered in cream sauce. The forty-eight-year-old journalist had had no previous interest in food—but when he returned to work after recovering from his hemorrhage, he started writing about exotic cookery.

Another hemorrhage patient experienced a similar foodie preoccupation, which prompted the doctors to start a three-year study. They found that, of more than seven hundred brain-hemorrhage patients, thirty-six developed what they named *gourmand syndrome.* They say in *Neurology* (1997, 48; 5:1185) that brain damage can sometimes unlock distant memories or unleash inhibitions, and it is possible that in some people it revives a buried passion for food.

Budding Disaster

Is your tongue about to get you into trouble? We all have different concentrations of tastebuds on our tongues, and a quarter of us are so-called supertasters, with highly sensitive palates.

This may sound great, but it can be to your peril, warn scientists at Wayne State University. Supertasters inhabit a "neon taste world" in which sensations such as bitterness are magnified. And this may put them off green vegetables, such as broccoli, and similar foods known to help protect against cancer. Dr. Linda Bartoshuk studied a group of men's colon cancer screening results and found a link between the number of precancerous colon polyps and the men's taste sensitivity.

There is some good news, though. Supertasters seem to have lower risk of heart disease, according to work done by Dr. Bartoshuk's colleague Valerie Duffy. She suggests in the *Journal of the American Dietetics Association* (2000, 100; 6:647) that this is probably because they tend to not like sweet and fatty foods.

Salt and Battery

Look out for those tiny batteries that come in watches, cameras, and telephones. In fact, look out for the bigger ones, too. There seems to be a strange human compulsion to swallow them.

Georgetown University's National Capital Poison Center reported 2,382 cases of adults and children swallowing batteries over a seven-year period in the journal *Pediatrics* (1992; 89:747–57). Most of them were button-sized batteries used in hearing aids and watches, but there were also much larger cylindrical cells.

The Center says that a surprisingly high number of adult patients have mistaken the batteries for pills. "One guy was walking down the street, reached into his pocket for something for a headache, and popped a battery in his mouth," says Georgetown's Dr. Toby Litovitz, the author of the study.

Another patient was taking a heart pill and changing her hearing-aid battery at the same time and mixed the two up. "She didn't realize what had happened until her hearing aid didn't work." (She can't have been able to hear her heart beating either, which must have been doubly distressing.)

It takes forty-eight hours for a battery to pass through the intestinal tract. The battery usually corrodes, leaking its alkaline fluids into the body. The poisons are often so diluted by body fluids that they cause little harm, though one in ten patients suffered symptoms such as vomiting and nausea.

The chief danger, says Dr. Litovitz, is that the button batteries can become lodged in the esophagus and have to be removed surgically. All six of the larger batteries, most of them size AAA, passed through the swallowers' bodies safely.

CHRISTIANS' BLOODY PERIL

Communion is at the heart of Christian fellowship, but that doesn't mean it is absolved from the normal rules of hygiene: so churchgoers should beware of poisoned chalices. Bernard Hudson, the head of microbiology and infectious diseases at Royal North Shore Hospital, Sydney, has warned the city's Anglicans to use individual cups to cut the infection risk.

The *Medical Post* (April 15, 2003) says that a report by Hudson dispels the notion that the wine in the chalice, which symbolizes Christ's blood, kills any infection. And, he adds, "It is not true to state that wiping the communion cup reduces the amount of infectious agent present to a level lower than the infectious dose."

Hudson has told the church it could be held liable if a parishioner contracts an infection such as the cold-sore virus or meningococcal septicemia from sharing saliva. He says, too, that dispensing bread with unwashed hands could spread diarrhea.

Passover Pass Out

The locusts, boils, and even the angel of death have passed over, but if you are an observant Jew, you now face a new threat to your children—from Passover lamps. A study of New Yorkers has discovered how Jewish toddlers risk poisoning from the lamp oil that illuminates holy days.

Dr. Robert J. Hoffman of Manhattan's Beth Israel Medical Center had noticed that on many Fridays when he worked at the city's Poison Control Center, urgent calls came in about children who had swallowed paraffin oil. "It turned out they were Jewish," Hoffman says. The accidents often happened during Sabbath, from sunset on Friday until sunset on Saturday, or on Jewish holidays such as Passover.

The oil can cause coughing, vomiting, and inflammation of the lungs. Hoffman found the cases shared a similar cause: "The lamps have a metal tube that serves as a wick. And when the lamp is not lit, the tube looks like a perfect straw to a child," he says.

The risk of paraffin-oil poisoning among the city's Orthodox Jewish children is about 370 times higher than in the general population, warns Hoffman's study in *Pediatrics* (2004, 113; 4:e377). He says that from 2000 to 2003 in New York, thirty-two out of forty-five oil-poisoning cases involved Orthodox Jewish children whose average age was under two.

Low-Cholesterol Killers?

So, you have paid heed to all the health warnings and cut your cholesterol intake. That may well have strongly reduced your chances of premature demise through heart attack, stroke, or high blood pressure. But it seems you may also have somewhat boosted your chances of dying by your own hand—or by someone else's.

The cholesterol debate is not as one-sided as you might think. Large-scale health promotion initiatives have shown that reducing cholesterol consumption lowers your chance of dying from cardiovascular disease, but a report in the *British Medical Journal* (1994, 309; 6942:421) says that if you cut your cholesterol intake, it could increase your chances of death through fatal accidents, suicide, and violence.

This has sparked controversy among researchers, who deny that such studies' conclusions are valid. But several explanations have been proposed for the strange phenomena. A California University, Los Angeles, study in the *Lancet* (1993, 341; 8837:75) reports a link between low cholesterol and increased incidence of depression among men over seventy. It suggests that this may be because low cholesterol levels shorten the amount of time the feel-good hormone serotonin is effective in the brain.

Some studies on mice show that cholesterol might help the central nervous system to suppress harmful behavioral impulses, while monkeys in zoos have been found to act abnormally aggressive when put on low-fat diets, according to a report in *Psychosomatic Medicine* (1991, 53; 6:634).

Men who murder in a fit of rage have also been found to show below-average cholesterol levels. A study in the

Lancet (1992, 340; 8826:995) suggests that some cholesterol-reducing drugs may increase aggressive behavior as a side effect, thus increasing patients' chances of getting into trouble.

But the criminal behavior seems to happen regardless of medication. University of California, Los Angeles, medical researchers compared the blood-cholesterol tests of 79,777 Swedes with their subsequent police records. They found that below-average cholesterol was strongly associated with criminal violence, even when the criminals were compared with people the same age and sex who had the same levels of education and drinking patterns, says a report in the *Journal of Psychiatric Research* (2000, 34; 4–5:301).

So the next time someone comes at you with a baseball bat, hand them a cupcake and a glass of whole milk.

Karaoke Victims

Barroom researchers have confirmed what many already suspect: karaoke singing can cause pain. Strenuous singing can injure the voice and increase the risk of deafness, according to two studies.

Researchers in Korea measured sound pressure levels during ballads and rock. They also measured each singer's hearing threshold levels before and after one hundred minutes of karaoke. Results showed that noise levels frequently exceeded the U.S. Occupational Safety and Health Administration's limit of 115 decibels, roughly equivalent to having a pneumatic drill going a meter away from your head.

"Up to eight decibels of significant hearing loss was found at the most important human hearing frequency band, after about two hours of karaoke. It may pose a serious threat," warns the study, in the *International Journal of Industrial Ergonomics* (2003, 31: 375–85).

In a second study, Hong Kong University researchers warn in the *Journal of Voice* (2003; 17:216–27) that karaoke singers risk committing vocal kamikaze. "As most of the karaoke singers have no formal training in singing, these amateur singers are more vulnerable to developing voice problems under these intensive singing activities," they discovered.

If you really want to trash your voice, hit the booze, avoid water, and go crazy. "Subjects who sang continuously without drinking water and taking rests showed significant changes in the jitter measure [i.e., warbling] and the highest pitch they could produce during singing," the researchers conclude.

Sid Vicious Syndrome

Harvard doctor Robert Caspari is no fan of rock music. He reports in the *New England Journal of Medicine* (1980, 303; 24:1420) how it can ruin your eyesight.

His patient, a healthy twenty-year-old man with a youthful taste in loud music, arrived at the doctor's complaining of redness in both eyes that had persisted for four days. On examination, Dr. Caspari found hemorrhaging in both eyes, but no immediate cause.

"After close questioning, the patient disclosed that on the night before the appearance of the redness he had been vigorously involved in a dance called the 'pogo' which is performed to New Wave music," says the doctor. "Reportedly this requires repeated bouncing movements for long periods of time."

Beaten by the Beat

Johns Hopkins Hospital doctors have identified a scourge of rhythm-crazy teens: *disco felons*. They write in the *New England Journal of Medicine* (1979, 301; 3:166) how they discovered it when treating a seventeen-year-old girl with an abscess on her middle finger. On close questioning, she said it had been caused by an infected crack in the skin—and the crack had been caused by constantly snapping her fingers in time to the music.

Disc Digit

Another recreational disease to afflict the middle digit is *Frisbee finger*. This emerged in the mid-seventies at the start of the Frisbee craze. Doctor Halley Faust of Philadelphia points out that the problem of infected finger cuts is greater among urban Frisbee throwers because the disc lands on hard surfaces, which makes the edges jagged. "The syndrome does occur if you overdo it with smooth-edged Frisbees as well, however, and should not be ruled out in subjects from more rural settings," he points out in the *New England Journal of Medicine* (1975, 293; 14:725).

HAVE YOU GOT THE BIG H?

Do you worry about being too worried about your health?

One classic definition of hypochondria is that it is "an irrational fear of disease so great that it disrupts normal living." Of course, that is clinically serious hypochondria rather than the lifestyle-level of daily health obsession we are nowadays all encouraged to feel. But you can find out your fear-factor by trying this Whiteley Index questionnaire.

The Whiteley Index is the standard self-test for hypochondria. For each question, circle the number that best describes how you feel.

1 = Not at all
2 = A little
3 = Moderately
4 = Quite a bit
5 = A great deal

1. Do you worry a lot about your health?

                               1   2   3   4   5

2. Do you think there is something seriously wrong with your body?

                               1   2   3   4   5

3. Is it hard for you to forget about yourself and to think about all sorts of other things?

1   2   3   4   5

4. If you feel ill and someone tells you that you are looking better, do you become annoyed?

1   2   3   4   5

5. Do you find that you are often aware of various things happening in your body?

1   2   3   4   5

6. Are you bothered by many aches and pains?

1   2   3   4   5

7. Are you afraid of illness?

1   2   3   4   5

8. Do you worry about your health more than most people?

1   2   3   4   5

9. Do you get the feeling that people are not taking your illnesses seriously?

1   2   3   4   5

10. Is it hard for you to believe your doctor when he tells you there is nothing to worry about?

1   2   3   4   5

11. Do you often worry about the possibility that you have a serious illness?

1   2   3   4   5

12. If a disease is brought to your attention (through
radio, TV, newspapers, or someone you know), do
you worry about getting it yourself?

1   2   3   4   5

13. Do you find that you are bothered by many different symptoms?

1   2   3   4   5

14. Do you often have the symptoms of a very serious
illness?

1   2   3   4   5

Add up the circled numbers. The higher your total,
the higher your chances of being excessively worried
about your health. There are no definite parameters in
the Whiteley Index, but if you score between 32 and 55
(or even more than that), you are generally considered a
hypochondriac. If you score between 14 and 28, you are
generally thought to be normal. These numbers are
merely indications, however, and people suffering from
depression can also often score high.

Doctors' Distraction

Joining the medical profession does not help to protect you from this crawling malaise. It makes it worse.
Oliver Howes, a psychiatrist at the Maudsley Hospital,
London, warns in the *Lancet* (1998, 351; 9112:1332) that
some studies have found that about 70 percent of medical
students suffer occasional bouts of hypochondriasis—
which is medically defined as a "persistent, unrealistic
preoccupation with the possibility of having a serious

disease." The definition goes on to say that
"common, normal sensations and appearances are often misinterpreted as abnormal and signs of disease."

Among the junior medics it is known as *medical studentitis,* and their health worries are often linked to the illness they happen to be studying at the time. Howes adds that other professionals reportedly prone to hypochondria are actors and musicians. Writers, politicians, and business types appear particularly high-risk, too.

Hypochondria— The Symptoms

Dr. F. E. Kenyon, a British psychiatrist who has spent most of his professional life working with hypochondriacs, says in the *British Journal of Psychiatry* (1976, 1; 29:1) that the most common places for imagined pains are the head and neck, followed by the abdomen and then the chest.

Head and neck complaints include dizziness, hearing one's own pulse at night, loss of hearing, a lump in the throat, throat clearing or cough, and floaters that drift across one's field of vision. Gastrointestinal complaints include indigestion in all its forms, followed by pains and bowel disorders.

Kenyon adds that chest complaints most usually concern palpitations, skipped heartbeats, pain on one side, racing pulse, inability to take a deep breath, involuntary sighing, and a sense of increased blood pressure. And from which side of the body do the mysterious pains emanate? Kenyon says that, inexplicably, around 70 percent of complaints are on the left.

BACK PAIN OR BRAIN PAIN?

Further evidence of the mind's ability to create specific phantom pains was unearthed by researchers at Stanford University School of Medicine in May 2004. They studied almost one hundred patients over four years and found that the ones who were considered to be depressed or neurotic at the beginning of psychological tests were nearly three times more likely to report back pain by the end of testing.

This may lead to many thousands of unnecessary surgical procedures, the researchers warn in *Spine* (2004; 29:1112), because only a quarter of the three hundred thousand spinal fusion operations performed each year in America are done for obvious reasons, such as removing deformities or tumors. Many back-pain patients, it seems, could have been better helped by psychological therapy.

And It's Contagious . . .

Hypochondria is contagious and can be transmitted from mothers to children, claim British psychologists.

Caroline Crane of Oxford University says women who haunt doctors with medically unexplained symptoms, such as irritable bowel syndrome (IBS), chronic headaches, and back pain, often display hypochondriacal symptoms such as an irrational fear of serious illnesses like cancer.

Crane's study of 227 mothers found that these hypochondriacal moms take their children to the doctor much more often than other mothers. The children also complain more frequently of stomach troubles, says the report in *The American Journal of Gastroenterology* (2004, 99; 4:694).

The study suggests that illness-obsessed parents over-react to their children's minor symptoms by marching them straight to the doctor. The children learn to imitate their parent's hypervigilance for minor symptoms and may also acquire their parent's particular illness—usually a disease believed to have a psychosomatic component, such as IBS or chronic fatigue syndrome.

But we should not condemn the mothers; the research says they seem to have been treated the same way by their own moms. The trouble could go back generations.

CLINIC CAPERS

If the illness doesn't get you, the medics might

Hospital—The Worst Place to Get Sick

One of the greatest dangers of being a hypochondriac is the chance that sooner or later some helpful medic will believe there may be something genuinely wrong with you physically. Then they'll send you for investigations and perhaps even an operation. And that's when you can really start worrying says a report in the *Journal of the American Medical Association* (2003, 290; 14:1868).

Some of the hazards of hospitalization are

- Serious blood infection after surgery: 22 percent of patients who contracted this died

- Rupture of a wound after surgery: nearly 10 percent died of the injury

- Other infections caused by medical care: these killed 4 percent of patients who contracted one

Medical injuries in hospitals claim more than 32,500 lives in the United States each year, according to a study of hospital-care complications led by Dr. Chunliu Zhan of the Agency for

Healthcare Research and Quality. Zhan, who spent two years identifying medical injuries in 7.5 million hospital cases from 2000, says that the safest procedure in the hospital is the delivery of a baby naturally, without the help of instruments. "Not too many people would die from those injuries."

Zhan's figures may, however, be a rather conservative estimate. *Effective Clinical Practice* (2000, 3; 6:277) says a report by the American Institute of Medicine on medical errors concludes that around 3.3 percent of hospital admissions result in a fatal error, and that half of these—between 44,000 and 98,000 patient deaths each year—are preventable. So according to this report, up to 268 people—the equivalent of an airliner load—are dying unnecessarily in America every day, thanks to doctors' mistakes.

First, Do Some Harm . . .

More cause to shun doctors: an anonymous survey of head and neck surgeons found that 45 percent admitted a medical error in their practice in the previous six months. More than a third of these had caused "major injury or harm," says the survey of twenty-five hundred members of the American Academy of Otolaryngology–Head and Neck Surgery. Four percent of the mistakes proved fatal.

According to *Laryngoscope* (2004, 114; 8:1322), the top five areas for error were:

- Technical mistakes during surgery (19 percent)

- Giving wrong medicines or the wrong doses (14 percent)

- Ordering wrong tests, not reading results, not acting on them (10 percent)

- Labs mislabeling specimens, losing them, or testing them wrongly (10 percent)

- Failing to plan operations properly (10 percent)

Tired Nurse curse

That nurse looking a bit stressed? Watch out. Nurses are three times more likely to make a mistake when working long shifts, says a Pennsylvania University study—and it warns that nurses are now working those long shifts 40 percent of the time.

The study, which tracked 393 nurses, found that about 40 percent of their shifts exceeded 12.5 hours—the point at which their errors really start to rack up. The nurses made 199 errors in the space of a month—that's around one mistake for every two staff.

Most of these involved giving patients the wrong drug or the wrong dose, or giving it later than it should have been administered. But the study, in the *Journal of Health Affairs* (2004, 23; 4:202), did not look at the impact all these blunders made on patients.

Oops, Now Where's That Clamp?

The most popular places in the body for surgeons to leave instruments inside you after operations are

- Abdomen or pelvis: 54 percent
- Vagina: 22 percent
- Chest: 7.4 percent
- Others, such as spinal canal, face, brain, and extremities: 17 percent

You are most at risk if you have emergency surgery or there's an unexpected change in your operation. In that case, the odds that the surgeons will leave something untoward inside your body are between four and nine times greater. Your risk also rises significantly if you are overweight: hefty people are more likely to have objects left inside because there is more room to lose things.

Sponges or instruments are left behind at least fifteen hundred times a year in the United States, say researchers led by Dr. Atul Gawande, a surgeon at Brigham and Women's Hospital in Boston. They say leaving objects behind is "an uncommon but dangerous error" that can lead to severe infections, organ damage, and sometimes even death.

In some cases surgical sponges (which are actually gauze pads) left in patients become embedded in tissue and are mistaken for tumors. As a result, patients have had parts of their intestines removed. Such errors occur in one out of every nine thousand to nineteen thousand operations where the body cavity is opened—about one case a year for a typical large hospital, says the report in the *New England Journal of Medicine* (2003, 348; 3:229).

In the language of medical journals, surgical tools sewn up inside people are not lost, forgotten, or left behind; rather, they are "retained." "It is kind of a euphe-

mism," Gawande says. "It implies a certain lack of responsibility, or that the instrument did it itself."

The profession has coined a word for a left-behind
surgical sponge: *gossypiboma,* from the Latin word *gossyp-
ium* for "cotton" and the Swahili *boma* for "place of con-
cealment."

House-Brick Hymen

It is not only medics who leave things in inappropriate
cavities. Doctors in the *Journal of the Indian Medical Association* (2002, 100; 11:671) report the case of a sixty-
year-old woman who turned up at a hospital reporting
constipation and pain in the lower abdomen. A rectal examination found a strange mass obstructing her bowel.
Careful manipulation removed the object from her vagina.
It measured 15 cm x 12 cm x 12 cm, and was a house
brick. The patient said it helped with her prolapse.

White-Coat Chaos

Professional incompetence is not the only medical
threat to patients. Simply wearing doctors' clothes can be a
danger. It is called the *white-coat effect.* People who get
panicked by health professionals give out strange diagnostic results, as shown by Toronto University researchers who
compared blood pressure readings taken by doctors in surgery with those taken by civilians outside the hospital.

They report in the *American Journal of Hypertension*
(2003, 16; 6:494) that the average readings taken by civilians were significantly lower than the doctors'—155
mmHg compared to 174 mmHg. Such a disparity can

mean the difference between "normal" and "troublesome."

But people whose blood pressure is liable to be sent soaring by the white-coat effect seem to have a right to be worried—they are significantly more liable to be female smokers with a family history of cardiovascular disease, says a study in the *British Journal of General Practice* (2003, 53; 495:790).

Blood-Pressure Blunders

There is one further reason why medics can send your blood pressure soaring. They often don't take the readings correctly. Nearly three quarters of healthcare workers fail to put your arm in the right position when taking blood-pressure readings, and this can make the result up to 10 percent higher, says a report in the *Annals of Internal Medicine* (January 8, 2004).

Investigators from the University of California, San Diego School of Medicine, and the Medical College of Wisconsin say that 73 percent of healthcare workers fail to use the proper arm position and blood-pressure cuff positions.

Just so you know, the researchers argue that the correct procedure is to position the patient's elbow at a right angle to the body, with the elbow flexed at heart level. In any other position, the reading can be so inaccurately high as to prompt doctors to start giving unnecessary treatment.

Math Disruption

Perhaps part of the problem is that doctors are not good with numbers. Statistical blunders are common in medical research reports—even when they are published in the most renowned medical journals. More than a third of the papers in the *British Medical Journal* and a quarter in *Nature* over a one-year period have at least one statistical error, say Spanish researchers.

They report in *BMC Medical Research Methodology* (2004; 4:13) that the obvious mistakes they found can significantly swerve the results of the research conclusions—thus misleading doctors about the best treatments to use. There may be many other mistakes, too, they add—but they can't find them because they would be buried deep in the doctors' early research calculations.

WEEKEND WIPEOUT

If you are planning an emergency hospitalization, avoid weekends. Patients admitted to surgical intensive care units on Saturday or Sunday are 30 percent more likely to die than those admitted on weekdays, researchers from a large teaching hospital have found. You need not worry, however, if it is a medical or multi-specialty intensive care unit, because they don't seem to suffer the weekend dip.

"We don't really know why surgical patients admitted on the weekend didn't fare as well," says Dr. Allen Ensminger of the Mayo Clinic in Minnesota. "Potentially there is a delay in seeking a surgeon for the patient admitted on the weekend," he told an American Thoracic

Society International Conference. Perhaps weekends are a good time to have a heart attack on the golf course instead.

Christmas Coronary

Christmas seems a bad time, too. Heart attack patients admitted to American hospitals during the winter holidays have higher mortality rates than those admitted during the rest of the year. Experts from Duke University Medical Center discovered from 134,000 medical records that during the holiday period, patients are more likely to receive second-rate drugs or surgery.

Why? It appears that the best doctors and surgeons have made sure that they get time off to spend with their families, leaving people unfortunate enough to get coronaries for Christmas in the hands of less able staff, says evidence presented to the American College of Cardiology.

Out-of-Hours Evil

Try to avoid having heart surgery outside of normal office hours. Coronary angioplasty is twice as likely to fail on heart attack patients if performed before 8 AM and after 6 PM. This time, though, it may not be the doctors' fault.

Dutch findings, in the *Journal of the American College of Cardiology* (2003, 41; 12:2138), suggest that the body's circadian rhythms have a strong impact on how well patients survive angioplasty operations. The results raise concern that the surgery results are worse for patients who have operations outside normal work hours. So are bodily rhythms at fault, or the fact that doctors don't like working antisocial hours?

In the same issue of the journal, doctors at the University of Massachusetts Medical School in Worcester say there is strong evidence that sleep deprivation impairs doctors' cognitive performance and motor function (i.e., it makes them dozy and clumsy).

Three Minutes—No, Two Minutes—to Live

Doctors may be able to predict times when they are not up to the job, but their colleagues who try to predict your death are seldom right. Researchers in the *British Medical Journal* (2003, 327; 7408:195) looked at the clinical prediction of survival and compared it with actual survival in eight studies for 1,563 patients.

The doctors, perhaps surprisingly, proved to be optimists. Maybe they have too much faith in their handiwork. While the medics predicted on average that patients had forty-two days to live, the average survival was only twenty-nine days. And although in a quarter of cases they were correct within seven days, more often than that they were off by at least four weeks.

The researchers, from Australia's Royal Prince Alfred Hospital in Camperdown, suggest that on average, doctors overestimate people's remaining lifespan by 30 percent. So if the doctor does announce that you have only three minutes to live, don't bother trying to boil an egg.

Body Talk, ER-Style

Want fast treatment in the emergency room? Don't cross your legs, suggest Micha Rapoport and colleagues at the Assaf Harofeb Medical Centre, Zerifin, Israel, in the *Lancet* (1995, 345; 8956:1060).

They say their experience of working in emergency rooms has taught them that when patients arrive on a stretcher with any of their limbs crossed—such as crossed ankles, crossed hands behind the neck, or hands folded across the stomach—they are "highly unlikely to have any acute condition, leaving ample time for tests and observation." The emergency-room medics take their relaxed postures as evidence that their problems are not urgent. Keep your legs apart—you'll get seen quicker.

Doctorspeak: The Terrible Truth

If you ever have the misfortune to witness a pair of hospital doctors talking across your bedridden body, listen carefully. That jumble of jargon and acronyms could reveal that they don't like you, or that your outlook is less than hopeful. Sincere condolences if you ever hear yourself described as CTP—that's "circling the plughole."

Doctors from hospitals in London and Cambridge compiled in *Ethics & Behavior* (2003, 13; 2:173) a list of slang terms used in medicine. Here they are, along with a few other old medical favorites:

Betty: Someone with diabetes
Cheerioma: Patient with a highly aggressive, malignant cancer
CLL: Chronic low life
Coffin dodger: Elderly patient
CTP: Circling the plughole

Departure lounge: Geriatric ward
Digging for worms: Varicose vein surgery
FLK: Funny-looking kid (in babies' notes)
Freud squad: Psychiatrists
Gassers: Anesthesiologists
GPO: Good for parts only
Guessing tube: Stethoscope
House red: Blood
LOBNH: Lights on but nobody home
Oligoneuronal: Of low intellect
Pest control: Term applied to psychiatrists by emergency-room workers
PFO: Pissed, fell over
PRATFO: Patient reassured and told to fuck off
Removal men: Department of care of elderly people
Rose cottage: Mortuary
Rule of five: If more than five orifices are obscured by plastic tubing, the patient's condition is considered critical
Slashers: General surgeons
Treat'n'street: Emergency-room's term for quick patient turnaround
TUBE: Totally unnecessary breast examination

Dammit, You Died of the Wrong Disease

Diagnoses are a wonderful thing—doctors have, with the benefit of science, technology, centuries of knowledge, and the investigative skill of an Agatha Christie detective, divined that you are *bona fide* ill. It is a shame then that their chances of getting the diagnosis right seem no better than about fifty-fifty.

That is the conclusion of researchers in Birmingham, United Kingdom, who examined the post-mortem notes of patients who had died in an intensive-care unit to discover what had actually killed them, compared with the doctors' original diagnoses.

They report in *Critical Care* (March 1, 2002) that their study of thirty-eight patients over a three-and-a-half-year period found that in 47 percent of the cases, doctors had missed the main cause of death. Only 42 percent of the patients' notes showed a complete agreement between the diagnosis and the post-mortem findings.

The doctors had most frequently failed to diagnose cancer, heart-valve failure, infections, and pulmonary embolism. Not exactly obscure stuff. And this was in people lying in beds for the critically ill. "Misdiagnosis may have led to unnecessary early death (if known for reversible causes) or unnecessary prolongation of life where terminal disease was present," the researchers conclude.

Prescription Perils

It is not only the medics who could get you. Prescribed drugs wreak their own havoc. In Australia, an estimated 6 percent of all hospital admissions and some 800 deaths a year are caused by people taking their medication incorrectly, reports the *Australian Health Review* (1998, 21; 4:260). We fret continually about the prospect of young people having access to recreational drugs, but rarely seem worried about telling confused and ill people to take jars of potentially lethal chemicals home.

HARD-HEARTED MEN

Any self-respecting hypochondriac is nigh certain to avoid donating blood, what with all those germs, and the lurking fear that you may somehow bleed to death. But keeping your plasma to yourself could increase your chance of arterial disease.

Kansas University Medical Center researchers claim that, unlike women, men don't get the chance to get potentially harmful iron out of their blood through menstruating. So males store it up—possibly harming their arteries. But, they report in the journal *Heart* (1997, 78; 2:188), donating blood twice a year can help solve the problem.

PET THERAPY

They don't just bite the hand that feeds

Eight Dogs, One Horse, One Donkey . . .

. . . Animals that were responsible for severely biting the penises of two men and eight boys who were rushed to São Paulo University Hospital between 1983 and 1999, as reported in the *Journal of Urology* (2000, 165; 1:80).

Love Lizard

Cuddly iguana? Some people swear the cold-blooded tongue-flickers are loving companions. But it can go too far. *The Journal of the American Association of Reptile Veterinarians* (Vol. 1, 1991) exposed eighteen cases of sexual assault by iguanas in American homes.

The pattern behind the attacks was so similar that it was highly unlikely to have been coincidence. In each case, the bond between animal and owner was unusually intimate. Some owners slept, showered, and ate with their pets.

In each case the animal was the sole iguana in the home, all attacks took place in the breeding season, and the offending reptile was male and sexually mature. The victims were female heads of the household, within childbearing age, and either menstruating or just about to start at the time of the attack.

The authors speculate that one or more components of human sexual pheromones are identical or similar to those occurring in iguanas. A cage, they suggest, is the answer.

BEWAREWOLF

Lycanthropy makes people believe they have been transformed into animals. It is sufficiently widespread to have spawned a self-help group in the United States called Werewolves Anonymous.

Yappy or Snappy?

Dogs kill 20 Americans each year and in-jure 585,000. The types of dogs most likely to bite, according to the Centers for Disease Control and Prevention, include

German shepherds
Chow chows
Collies
Male or unneutered dogs
Dogs belonging to a household with children
Dogs chained up in a yard.

The safest breeds, according to *Pediatrics* (June 1994), are

Golden retriever
Standard poodle

Nice Doggie . . . er

The fatal dog-bite attack league table for the quarter-century from 1979 to 1998, compiled for the *Journal of the American Veterinary Medical Association* (2000, 217; 6:836), shows that of the top human-killing breeds, more than half were pit-bull types or rottweilers.

But think also *location, leash, location*: 58 percent involved unrestrained dogs on their owners' property 24 percent involved unrestrained dogs off their owners' property; and 17 percent involved restrained dogs on their owners' property.

Feline Fear Factor

You are much safer with a cat. But somehow it may be much more traumatic to be viciously mauled by a mewling assailant called Fluffy or Tinkerbell. U.K. Department of Health figures show that eighteen thousand people were injured in cat-related incidents in the year 2002 alone.

And when Kitty gets vicious, things quickly go all Stephen King. Pensioner Leila Johnstone, sixty-six, was asleep when her puss, Susie, launched a frenzied attack. It sank its claws into Johnstone's forehead and ripped her arm through to the bone. Johnstone thinks her pet may have been spooked by a ginger tomcat sitting outside her flat.

"I woke up with this black thing hanging on to me. I fought her but she still clung on. I didn't know what was happening and I was terrified. There was blood everywhere and I thought I was done for," she tells the *Scottish Daily Record* (August 29, 1997).

Johnstone, of Glasgow, Scotland, managed to break free but Susie chased her and gouged her leg before Johnstone shut her in the room. Johnstone was then rushed to the hospital. "I still don't feel right," she told the *Record*. "I'm feeling sick and dizzy all the time. And I can't believe the cat did this. I'm just glad it didn't happen to any of my grandchildren."

Susie the cat was put down.

Edna Brown, eighty-three, was mauled so badly by her tabby cat called McGuinty that she needed twenty-seven stitches. Police who attended the incident at Elmira told the *Toronto Star* (August 11, 2000) they had seen less blood at murder scenes.

"He just grabbed my legs," Brown says of her gray-and-white assailant. "I pulled him off and I threw him into the corner and then he attacked again. He wouldn't let go."

Brown managed to shove the hissing pet into her apartment and ran out. She then collapsed, the blood from her wounded ankles and right arm pouring down the hallway steps. "I don't know why he attacked me. We were best of friends," she says.

Dr. Gerard Hess of the local Kitchener-Waterloo Humane Society tells the paper it is not uncommon for cats to turn on their owners. He gets such reports about once a month.

Just about anything, it seems, can spark cat rage. When Cocoa Puff, a four-year-old Siamese, attacked a family and sent them fleeing from their home, jealousy was blamed as the motive. The frenzy left Laurel Mancini, her husband, and her children bleeding from deep scratches and bites. The family told the *Calgary Sun* (May 15, 2002) they believe the cat became agitated after the Mancini family's babysitter admired their new kitten. "The cat just snapped," says Robert Mancini.

Gerard Daigle, eighty, lost half a liter of blood and required stitches after his cat, Touti, launched a frenzied attack, reports Australia's *Gold Coast Bulletin* (July 14, 2001). The provocation? Daigle was giving his pet parrot a shower when he inadvertently sprayed Touti the cat with water.

Who Gets Bit

Men are at greater risk of being bitten by dogs, adult women by cats, and young girls by horses, a two-year emergency-room study in Norway reveals in *Tidsskr Nor Laegeforen* (1998, 118; 17:2614).

With Pets, Watch What You Pat

Household cats and dogs can harbor salmonella, campylobacter, and other stomach-poisoning bacteria. Their paws can carry high levels of multiresistant staphylococcus aureus (MRSA).

Rabbits can spread listeriosis, salmonella, and even bubonic plague.

Horses can carry Lyme disease, salmonella, and encephalitis.

Around 38 percent of tortoises are infected with salmonella.

Town pigeons can spread at least ten serious infectious diseases, from mild food poisoning to viral encephalitis.

*Sources: Dr. Robert Baker, research fellow in infectious diseases at the Centre for Infectious Diseases, London, England (*Independent, *October 14, 1999). International Scientific Forum on Home Hygiene (2002).*

HISTORY OF THE BIG H

From Greek ribs to a possible cure

It is easy to believe hypochondria is so deeply wired into the human brain that it has always been with us—and always will be. According to the writer Aldous Huxley: "Directly or indirectly, most of our physical ailments and disabilities are due to worry and craving. We worry and crave ourselves into high blood pressure, heart disease, tuberculosis, peptic ulcer, low resistance to infection, neurasthenia, sexual aberrations, insanity, suicide. Not to mention the rest."

Perhaps that's a bit strong, but it is reckoned that hypochondriac patients form between 4 percent and 6 percent of the average community doctor's workload, says Dr. Brian Fallon, an associate professor of psychiatry at Columbia University in New York and coauthor of *Phantom Illness: Shattering the Myths of Hypochondria*. Other studies put the figure even higher.

But where did hypochondria come from? I like to imagine that the condition stretches back to our early hunter-gatherer ancestors, recently down from the trees and finding life on the ground so fraught that it has got them complaining of flint-napper's elbow and post-Jurassic stress disorder. The H word itself comes somewhat later—courtesy of the ancient Greeks. It derives from *hypochondrium* and refers to a specific place in the body, notably *hypo* (under) and *chondros* (the cartilage of the ribs). This anatomical description seems first to have been used by Hippocrates in 4 B.C.

Greek Health Freak

Galen of Pergamon used it to describe stomach disorders and, because the Greeks believed abdominal organs were the source of disordered emotions, hypochondrium started to take on its second, more popular meaning—disease obsession—around A.D. 2. For the next four hundred years its best-loved attributes were added: pre-occupation with disease, inexplicable periods of anxiety, and nightmares. The early doctors also linked it to melancholia, which may be a wise deduction—modern medical wisdom says many hypochondriacal patients may also be clinically depressed.

In seventeenth-century Europe, hypochondria started to be used to describe a depressive disorder that was characterized by indigestion and vague whiny pains. Leeches, those aspirins of the Middle Ages, were the preferred treatment. One can imagine the good apothecary scribbling busily on a parchment in order to avoid meeting the eyes of his persistently incurable patient and saying, "Just take two leeches a day, and if it doesn't clear up in a fortnight, come back and see me again."

Hip to Be Hyp

A good dose of leeching should have been enough to deter any hypochondriac from complaining too loudly, but instead the condition actually became fashionable across pestilence-ridden Renaissance Europe. For this, says Susan Baur, the author of *Hypochondria: Woeful Imaginings,* you can blame the Italian arty in-crowd. They threw out the age-old convention that rudely wholesome gladiator types were the guys to have at your party. Instead, they invented the idea that pale neurotics were interesting and cool, thus anticipating the New York punk scene by three hundred years and setting up the classic jock vs. nerd confrontation central to any frat-house movie.

The English Malady

The fashion for writhingly neurotic screwups rapidly spread northward to its fog-bound natural incubator—Britain. In 1733, George Cheyne, a pop doctor of the period, wrote the early hypochondriac's handbook, *The English Malady: a treatise of nervous diseases of all kinds, as spleen, vapours, lowness of spirits, hypochondriacal and hysterical distempers, etc.* Cheyne blamed the condition on "The moisture of our air, the variableness of our weather, the richness and heaviness of our food, the wealth and abundance of the inhabitants, the inactivity and sedentary occupations of the better sort (among whom this evil mostly rages) and the humor of living in great, populous and consequently unhealthy towns."

Cheyne declared that roughly one third of his countrymen suffered from hypochondria and hysteria. He added that the disease tended to afflict persons of greater intelligence and upper social class, and the condition became so chic that it came to be called "hyp." An anxious, gloomy temperament became both a sign of high intelligence and a must-have fashion accessory. The writers

Boswell and Johnson were among the hippest of the hyppies.

Victorian Vice

It was not until the following century, though, that hypochondria came to be narrowly defined as an excessive fear of illness. Historians speculate that the morbid Victorian obsession with sickness grew in step with the development of medical science, which helpfully kept discovering more and more new illnesses and health threats for us all to worry about—while technology, sanitation, and medical advances actually made huge leaps in making our lives far safer than ever before.

Hypochondria cured?

Psychologists have announced some potentially devastating news for hypochondriacs—or at least for the medics, therapists, life gurus, and pharmaceutical companies that profit from them: there may be a cure for hypochondria (or what in modern polite-speak is increasingly being defined as "health anxiety").

Arthur J. Barsky, previously cited in this book for his work on the nocebo effect (see page 21), reports in March 2004 that cognitive behavioral therapy can significantly alleviate hypochondriacal fears. He and colleagues at the Brigham and Women's Hospital and the Harvard Medical School, Boston, gave six weeks' worth of ninety-minute psychotherapy sessions to patients whose reported medical symptoms could not be explained by any real illness.

Barsky reports in the *Journal of the American Medical*

Association (2004, 291; 12:1464) that he studied 187 hypochondriacal patients for a year: 102 were given psychotherapy, while the rest were run through the medical system. Unfortunately, a quarter of the psychotherapy patients left the program as soon as they learned it was offering a mental rather than physical cure for the problems they perceived. "Most hypochondriac people never will go to a psychiatrist," says Barsky. "They will say, 'I don't need to talk about this, I need somebody to stick a biopsy needle in my liver, I need that CAT scan repeated.'"

Nevertheless, those who stuck with the six psychotherapy sessions explored the five factors that can lead people to blow their bodily symptoms out of all proportion and then convince themselves they have a serious disease. The factors are: their hypervigilance about bodily functions; their beliefs about what causes their apparent symptoms; their mood; the circumstances that start them obsessing; and their need to behave like sick people. The sessions also encouraged patients to stop habits that worsen their symptoms, such as Googling for disease information on the internet, browsing newspaper obituaries, and reading books like this one.

A year after the weekly ninety-minute sessions, Barsky reports that almost 57 percent of the patients had "significantly lower levels of hypochondriacal symptoms, beliefs, and attitudes and health-related anxiety." That represents a reasonably encouraging increase over the 32 percent of hypochondriacal patients whose lives improved after going through the normal medical system—though in both sets of patients, their actual physical symptoms did not go away. But then we all get back tweaks, stomach growls, headaches, and so on.

It seems that this intensive approach could therefore work for a sizable number of people whose hypochondria is so severe it can wreck their lives. And it certainly seems to work much better than the traditional medical response: either ignore them or give them a tablet—or even an operation—to make them go away.

On the Other Hand . . .

Individuals might be curable. But what about a wholesale remedy for today's hypochondriacal society? Would Western civilization be able to carry on without empty threats to obsess about? We might simply dance free of our old fearful shackles and live long lives of stressless joy. Given Homo sapien's innate drive to fixate on threat and danger, it seems far more likely that we would end up like the urban myth about hedgehogs, which says that if you rid them of their fleas, they start to suffer withdrawal symptoms.

A constant barrage of newly reported threats to our well-being does rather jazz up our sometimes mundane lives and distract us from difficult spiritual questions such as that old nagger, What is the meaning of it all? Orwell's *1984* featured global war as a constant distractor and motivator. We have our health to worry about. Shame it makes us ill.

WORLD OF WORK

Good day at the office, Dear?

Death by Corrupt Colleagues

Better hope your coworkers and organization are all free of scandal. If they aren't, your chances of killing yourself could leap.

It's called *Di Pietro syndrome* and was identified after mass media coverage of a government bribes case in Italy at the end of the 1980s caused widespread suspicion of people who worked in public services. This, say researchers at Policinico Hospital, Milan, exacerbated pre-existing psychiatric problems in public administrators and workers, as shown by the suicide of five local council managers after they were interviewed by investigators.

One, a thirty-five-year-old health administrator in a Milanese hospital, jumped in front of a train. He survived, and told how he had developed delusions, anxiety and depression, and guilt about imagined—and wholly nonexistent—shortcomings in his work performance, after he had read about the arrest of managers in the city's healthcare system. The irrational fear of being discovered and jailed prompted the suicide attempt, reports the *Psychiatric Bulletin* (1993, 17; 4:246).

Hairdresser's Nipple

Beware if you are a woman and a hairdresser. It may not be just the customers' generosity that leads you to getting bigger tips. Doctors at the Queen Elizabeth Hospital, England, who treated a female patient for painful breast infections have reported the first known case of hairdresser's nipple in the *British Medical Journal* (1988, 297; 6664:1641).

They discovered the phenomenon when they found that sharp little male hairs had penetrated her areolas, causing them to become infected and inflamed. This, they concluded, had been caused by her brushing too closely against her clients, whose coarse stubble had penetrated her clothes.

THIS JOB KILLS ME

The top professions for suicide risk are

- Dentists (poisoning)

- Vets (poisoning)

- Farmers (guns)

If you are male, single, or widowed and between ages fifteen and forty-four, then you are in the highest risk group for killing yourself, says the U.K. government report, *Trends in Suicide in England and Wales, 1982–96 Office of National Statistics.*

If you do plan on ending it all, be warned that the old hosepipe-from-the-exhaust method is out of fashion—

and less effective than ever. The report says the fall in suicides from poisoning by motor vehicle exhaust gas since the early 1990s is due to the growing number of cars fitted with catalytic converters.

Muse Misery

Tortured artists have a grim time of it. But writers and painters have much higher rates of suicide than musicians. Perhaps the tunes keep your spirits high, suggest Italian researchers in *Psychological Report* (2001, 89; 3:719).

Seasonal Suicide

Getting out in the fresh air might cheer you up, but then again, working in the great outdoors seems to have a strange seasonal effect on employees' suicide rates.

Finnish psychiatrists have discovered that farmers and forestry workers kill themselves most in the cheerful countryside season of spring and commit the fewest suicides in dismal, cold winter. People who work indoors kill themselves most frequently in summer, they report in the *Journal of Affective Disorders* (2002, 70; 2:197) Those open office windows must sometimes look too tempting.

Business Travel Trauma

Jet setting is not all glamour—in fact, those tempting overseas trips may prove rather sickening for travelers and their stay-at-home spouses.

Researchers at the World Bank in Washington, D.C., studied more than ten thousand of their staff to see if global travel harmed their health. The results show that their rates of health-insurance claims are significantly higher than nontraveling staff.

The biggest problem is psychological disorders, followed by infections—and the more the employees travel, the more problems they have. Interestingly, though, while male business travelers report an 80 percent increase in illnesses, the women's ill-health rate is up by only 18 percent, says the research in *Occupational and Environmental Medicine* (1997, 54; 7:499).

But it is not only the travelers who suffer. If you are the spouse of a global business-trotter, your chances of falling ill also increase considerably, the researchers revealed in the same publication (2002, 59; 3:175). Business-trippers' husbands and wives are 16 percent more likely to need medical treatment for physical and mental illness, their study finds.

The spouses suffer three times the rate of stress-related psychological disorders seen in nontravelers' partners. And they also have a much higher rate of skin and stomach diseases—which may indicate that the travelers bring home some unfortunate souvenirs. What the World Bank occupational health researchers could not explain, however, is why travelers' spouses also develop a significantly higher number of cancers.

Downshift Disaster

Tempted by the dream of dropping out of the promotion race to pursue a more balanced life? Perhaps you should think again. Folk wisdom might believe that high-status, stressed business leaders are heading for an early demise. But it's the underdog that gets it, says Professor Robert Evans of British Columbia University.

A study of civil servants working at the heart of the British government has found that people at the bottom of the hierarchy consistently die younger than those at the top, and not because they were poorer or had less apparently healthy lifestyles. Over ten years, those in the lowest grades had three times as great a likelihood of dying as those at the top.

Similar patterns were found among wild baboons in the Serengeti in East Africa. Social strain is apparently to blame. "What really bothers subordinates is not being attacked by a leopard, or even worrying about being attacked by a leopard," Evans told the British Association's science festival in September 1994. "It is being yawned at by a higher-ranking male at a distance of 3 feet."

From the Serengeti to the Houses of Parliament and Capitol Hill, the professor perceives a similar effect, where being an underling causes hormonal stress that could help explain the increased incidence of disease. "What seems to be harmful is the chronic strain that comes from being subjected to frequent and unpredictable attack, both physical and particularly psychological," he says.

Supervisor Stroke

If the slacking doesn't get you, your boss might. Working under someone you consider to be an unfair manager could increase your risk of heart attack or stroke, claims a study of healthcare workers. Your blood pressure really does go up if you work for someone considered routinely unreasonable, claims this experiment involving female healthcare assistants.

The assistants with duff supervisors had 15 mmHg higher systolic and 7 mmHg higher diastolic blood pressure than colleagues who felt more fairly managed. How bad is that? An increase of 10 mmHg in systolic and 5 mmHg in diastolic blood pressure is associated with a 16 percent increased risk of coronary heart disease and a 38 percent increased risk of stroke, says the report, in the *Journal of Occupational and Environmental Medicine* (2003, 60; 7:468).

The U.K. research authors, at Buckinghamshire Chilterns University College's Department of Human Sciences, say creating happier workplaces could prove a cheap way of cutting cardiovascular disorders. But then the employees end up living long enough to start draining the company pension fund.

Maimed by Boredom

Studies at the University of Northumbria, England, have found that bored people have more sick days off than any other group.

Maybe they are just slackers who would rather feed the ducks than sit shifting paper around their desks. Or perhaps they are suffering from *underload syndrome*. Dr. Martyn Dyer-Smith, a psychologist, warns, "Boredom has exactly the same effect on the body as stress. People who are normally busy can become ill when they don't have enough to do, because it sends their levels of stress hormones shooting up."

The *Sunday Times* (February 2, 2003) listed the most

common health complaints triggered by underload syndrome—headaches, fatigue, and recurrent infections, as well as mild depression. It added, "Research shows that highly strung people and those who are always on the go are most at risk. High-flyers are particularly vulnerable because they have perfected their skills and therefore are able to perform their jobs with little effort."

Cling-on Crisis

Maybe you should hang on to your job throughout the economic storms and tempests known as recession and lay-offs. At least it will be exciting. But then again, surviving a downturn with your career intact may only serve to accelerate your appointment with death.

Seven-and-a-half years after a big round of recessionary cutbacks in Finnish councils, statisticians examined the fates of 22,430 council employees who had managed to keep their full-time jobs. The figures showed their death rates from heart attacks and strokes had doubled, particularly in the first four years—the period when people are most likely to die after an event that causes shock or grief—after the lay-offs.

The study, led by the Finnish Institute of Occupational Health in four towns in Finland—Espoo, Turku, Vantaa, and Raisio—suggests the increased death rates are due to the fact that the staff who hung on to their jobs had to work harder to ensure their organizations provided the same level of service.

At the same time they were left feeling very insecure about their employment prospects. The remaining workers also felt they did not have much control over their careers. If you subject rats in a lab to those types of stresses, they soon fall over.

If it is any consolation, the *British Medical Journal* report (2004, 328; 7439:555) points out that the risk of cardiovascular death among the people who had been laid off was even higher than that among those who kept their jobs. Either way, human beings don't seem well built to survive economic downturns.

Boom of Doom

You might expect that economic good news would boost your health, wealth, and happiness. But Swedish research shows it can land you in the hospital. Sickness and hospital claims jump if the company you work for starts to expand.

The study, in the *Lancet* (2004, 363; 9416:1193), says that when companies increase their workforce by 18 percent or more, the long-term absence from sickness among existing staff rises significantly.

Their examination of more than twenty-four thousand individual cases from Swedish work surveys from 1989 to 1999 found that women working in the public sector are most at risk of *upsizing trauma*. The surprised researchers speculate that office "growing pains" such as organizational instability, difficulty finding decent new employees, and longer lines in the cafeteria may increase existing workers' stress.

OFFICE SMOG

You might have paused to worry about the ozone that old fax machines puff out, but have you ever thought about the dust storms of dead skin, crumbling cosmetics, scalp creatures, hair yeasts, and foot fungi that our office colleagues create? Not to mention dust mites' debris.

David Bodanis, a social theory lecturer at Oxford University, warns that vacuuming office carpets flings up colonies of microscopic dust mites living there. The mites' anal pellets shatter as they get pulled into the vacuum cleaner, only to be propelled as fragments into the air. The pellets contain digestive enzymes from the mites' guts, which can irritate many workers' eyes and lungs.

What's more, your fellow workers are constantly sloughing off bits of their bodies, says Bodanis, the author of *The Secret Garden* and *The Secret House*. Cosmetics crumble and talc slabs tear off and float loose. Nail polish evaporates and clothing fibers scrape away. We bring other things into the office from home: soil fragments, bits of pet fur, broken-off leaf hairs, and large numbers of tiny, amputated insect limbs.

We shed many thousands of skin flakes a minute. Sweat particles and leftover soap fragments work through small gaps in our clothes. Then there are scalp creatures, hair yeasts, and often even foot and other fungi. There is also all the stagnant carbon dioxide we breathe out, as well as the streams of methane and hydrogen sulphide bubbles we vent. Heat from our blood vessels provides constant gusts of warm air that rise from our bodies, lifting chunks of clothing, skin, and cosmetics up to ceiling height.

We eject, on average, about two-and-a-half saliva droplets per word, so a few hours of cross-desk chatting at a steady thirty words per minute sling out fifteen thousand droplets per person. These may spend an hour or more bobbing around before sinking. A number will have more dangerous types of staphylococci, and if there's been a sneeze anywhere within yards of you, it will eject a million or more droplets—viruses in them can float around, remaining alive, for thirty minutes or more.

Ever thought about working from home?

Price of Flame

Running away to the circus may seem the answer. All that glamour, the sawdust, the tigers, and the trapeze acts—and one or two personal perils you may not have considered.

Fire-eating, for example. Once you've got the hang of it, the act should be straightforward. Swiss medics, however, warn that performers run a high risk of hydrocarbon pneumonitis—or as the doctors from the Medizinische Klinik, Bezirksspital Dornach, prefer to call it, *fire-eater's lung.*

This is caused by inhaling petrol fumes too often and can lead to coughs, breathing trouble, chest pains, and fever, they report in the *Schweiz Medizinische Wochenschrift* (1994, 5; 124(9):362). The patient they studied also developed a nasty chest infection and was seriously ill for three weeks. He recovered fully two months later, but maybe he moved on to something healthier, such as lion-taming, after that.

Early Grave Please, Driver

Driving a bus or taxi boosts your risk of heart attack, claim Swedish researchers.

Professional drivers are also more likely to smoke and be overweight, but the increased risk could not be explained by these or other known risk factors, says Dr. Carolina Bigert of Karolinska Hospital in Sweden.

Bus drivers are more than twice as likely to have a heart attack as men who never worked as professional drivers. Taxi drivers' risk is only slightly lower, says the report in *Epidemiology* (2003, 14; 3:333).

Dr. Bigert says this may be due to stress, but she isn't sure.

PLANET PANIC

It's a nasty old world out there

Fatal Magnetic Attraction

The Earth's magnetic field might be threatening your life.

Despite the wealth of knowledge built up by the world's cardiologists, nearly a third of heart-related deaths still cannot be explained by known risk factors, argue Israeli doctors. So they looked skyward and earthward to examine if cardiac deaths are related to sunspots, changes in solar radiation, or changes in Earth's magnetic activity.

They used statistics of death rates among people in Lithuania over a ten-year period and claim they found that the total monthly number of heart fatalities was "significantly linked" with levels of activity in Earth's geomagnetic field. This, they add, was particularly true among people between ages sixty-five and seventy-four.

We should take heart from one piece of good news, though: the team from Rabin Medical Centre reports in *Biomedical Pharmacotherapy* (2002, 56; 2:301s) that accident levels go down when sunspots are more active.

Motor Misery

Perhaps it is not planet Earth's magnetic effect that causes heart deaths. Italian researchers suggest it could be the fault of electric fields caused by something much more mundane.

Rome University physicians say that mortality figures from hospitals in St. Petersburg, Russia, show that heart-attack death rates fall by one-and-a-quarter times on weekends. They looked for correlations with electric storms on Earth and in space, and found no link.

Instead, they suggest in *Biofizika* (1998, 43; 4:623) that our exposure to trains' and trams' electric motors when commuting to work may expose us to low-frequency magnetic fields that are powerful enough to bring our tickers to an unscheduled halt.

Star Stricken

Too down to earth? Let's go up into the heavens: perhaps the puppet-strings of our fates are being tugged by distant galaxies. Our star signs can determine our deaths, warn astrologists.

A study of local death records by Liverpool University in *Medical Science Law* (2003, 43; 2:111) claims that people born under the sign of Virgo have the highest risk of committing suicide by hanging themselves.

People born under summer-month star signs have the highest chance of suffering any kind of violent death, says the report. But Sagittarians and Scorpions can take heart—they are the Zodiac signs with the least danger of killing themselves.

On the other hand, Auburn University sociologists say in *Perception and Motor Skills* (1988, 66; 2:461) that only those born under the most negative sign of Pisces have a significantly raised risk of feeling suicidal.

In another study, the Manchester University Management School marketing lecturer, Vincent-Wayne Mitchell, says that U.K. government statistics on population behavior show that men's health risks are related to their birth signs.

Mitchell says that men born under Aries, Aquarius, and Pisces are more likely to smoke, and he claims this is because they are less open to persuasion about health risks. Men with more outgoing star signs, such as Gemini, are more likely to have an alcohol problem, because they think drinking is sociable, he says in the *Journal of Consumer Marketing* (1997, 14; 2:113).

Moon Mania

Werewolves are the least of your worries from lunar influence. The full moon increases your chance of being assaulted or poisoned, committing suicide, being hospitalized for psychiatric disorders—or getting bitten by dogs.

Doctors studied crime patterns over a 5,478-day period from January 1978 to December 1982 in three towns in India—one rural, one urban, and one industrial. They found that the mean crime rate was at its lowest seven days after a full moon, when 0.4 crimes were reported per day. On the full-moon day it shot up to an average of 1.4 crimes.

The study's authors, from Patna Medical College in India, are particularly interested in cases of poisoning, and suggest that, "The increased incidence of crimes on full-moon days may be due to 'human tidal waves' caused by the gravitational pull of the moon."

How so? They say that the human body is around 50 percent to 60 percent water, and that the full moon's gravitational pull creates a physical tide in people. And at high tide, the researchers argue, people tend to get out of hand and start dropping poison into the curries of people they don't like.

Their article, in the *British Medical Journal* (1984, 289; 6460:1789), cites previous research in the *Psychological Report* showing that suicides and psychiatric admissions rise at full moons, and a study in the *Journal of Clinical Psychiatry* which reports that aggressive incidents also multiply. Full moons do, however, seem to prompt a reduction in the number of women attempting to poison themselves, say toxicologists in the *Medical Journal of Australia* (1993, 159; 11–12:786). It is the new moon that causes problems—self-poisoning cases go up by a quarter, they report.

This might all sound like lunacy, but the research is further supported by Dr. Peter Perkins, a general practitioner in Bournemouth, England, in the *Journal of Epidemiology and Community Health* (1994, 48; 3:323). He says his interviews with seventy-nine general practitioners show their emergency calls increase by 3 percent when there is a full moon, and drop to 6 percent below average when there is a new moon. A decade previously, similar research showed a link between full moons and urinary retention in men with prostate trouble.

Then there is a report in *Family Practitioner* (2000, 17; 6:472), where doctors at the Nuffield Institute for Health's Center for Research in Primary Care studied the "so-called Transylvania hypothesis," and found a 3.6 percent increase in people coming to GP surgeries at full moons—which they describe as "small but statistically significant."

Doctors at the Institute of Preventive and Clinical Medicine in Bratislava, Slovakia, say their study of gout attacks between 1972 and 1994 shows that they peak under both new and full moons. They report in *Medical Hypotheses* (2000, 55; 1:24) that they have also seen similar patterns with bronchial asthma in children.

Barking Mad

It is not just humans who act strange under full moons, say doctors in northern England who studied the pattern of patients coming into the emergency room at the Bradford Royal Infirmary between 1997 and 1999. In all, 1,621 new patients had been bitten by animals— 1,541 dog bites, 56 cat bites, 13 horse bites, and 11 rat bites.

The lowest day for bites was the seventh day after a full moon, where 41 bite victims were admitted over ten lunar cycles. The highest was the full moon, when 119 victims came into the hospital. "The rise in incidence seemed to accelerate a few days before a full moon, peaking sharply on the day of a full moon before falling away rapidly," says the report in the *British Medical Journal* (2000, 321; 7276:1559).

Ill Winds

The *Lancet* in 2000 reports that the weather, as well as the moon, may have an important influence on health emergencies. In 1999, it says, the number of hospital admissions due to acute asthma attacks tended to rise after there had been a thunderstorm. It speculates that this may be due to a combination of high temperature, high humidity, high pollen counts, and poor air quality.

Manure Mayhem

Here's a danger that is much more down to earth: landing in shit can be lethal. Doctors at the Kantonsspital, St. Gallen, Switzerland, warn anyone fancying a quiet life in the countryside that farm manure stores can be lethal traps. They report that a total of forty-nine people had been killed in sixty-one major manure-related accidents in Switzerland.

Twelve of these victims were brave people who had dived into manure tanks in attempts to rescue colleagues who had become trapped there. The majority of deaths described in the *International Journal of Occupational Health* (1999, 5; 3:177) had been caused by inhaling manure gas, but eleven people had fallen into the stuff and drowned, while another six had been killed by methane explosions.

Hayfever? That's Nothing

Allergies are all the rage. But they can, it seems, get much wilder than simply making you sneeze. Take Josephine Hughes, who said she is so sensitive to animals that she can sense cats and dogs passing outside her home. "I can smell a cat walking across the street," Hughes, a former school cafeteria worker, told the *San*

Francisco Chronicle (February 27, 1990). "I can be sleeping and I wake up feeling cat hairs in my throat. If a dog goes by, it's like I have a clothes pin over my nose."

Jenny Wyatt who lives in Surrey, England, says she is allergic to electricity. "It started in 1999 when my family bought a fridge-freezer and I started experiencing strange symptoms," she says. "Within minutes of walking into the kitchen I'd feel dizzy and I had mood swings—bursting into tears and feeling depressed."

Wyatt says she had contracted chronic fatigue syndrome after having the flu in 1995, and a couple of years later developed food and chemical sensitivities. She seemed to be stabilizing when the new symptoms appeared. She tells the *Independent on Sunday* (September 2, 2001) that she wears magnetic insoles, cooks on a portable gas stove, and can stand only muted lighting— she often uses candles.

Tony Doherty of Northern Ireland was saved from a jail sentence in 1986 after a court accepted his claim that he was violently allergic to potatoes. The full extent of his allergy became clear only after he ate two packets of potato crisps and then attempted to strangle his father with a tie. The problem had not been identified before the court case. The twenty-one-year-old County Antrim man was warned to stay away from potatoes, says the *Courier Mail* (September 22, 1986).

Betty Napiers told the *Orlando Sentinel* (December 18, 1994) that she is allergic to the modern world, having to wear a purple-and-yellow gas mask on visits to her local shopping mall because exposure to makeup, aftershaves, suburban lawns, carpets, or stores' electronics sections made her feel sick and disoriented and suffer burning sensations in her skin. Napiers said she suffers from multiple chemical sensitivity (MCS), an illness first reported in America. According to Peter Radetsky, the author of *Allergic to the 20ᵗʰ Century,* more than 2.5 million Americans suffer from MCS.

Allergic to Everything

Multiple chemical sensitivity is a condition characterized by a gamut of allergic reactions. It is claimed to be a dysfunction of the nervous system caused by an overload of offending agents. Many sufferers claim it has ruined their lives. One female sufferer is reported to hang her mail on a clothesline for two weeks to allow it to "detoxify" before she can read it.

A paper from the Chemical Injury Information Network lists more than a hundred symptoms that may result from MCS. These include sneezing, itching, twitching, hoarseness, earache, high or low blood pressure, sore muscles, cramps, frequent urination, PMS, lower backache, nausea, belching, constipation, hunger, thirst, headaches, apathy, forgetfulness, insomnia, depression, heat sensitivity, cold sensitivity, stiffness, swelling, pain in the neck, agitation, and genital sweating.

The bottom of the page adds: "Unfortunately this is not a complete list of symptoms."

Loud Shirt Sensitivity

The allergy phenomenon has been growing since the 1950s, when Amelia Nathan Hill set up Action Against Allergies in America and persuaded millions of people that their headaches, fatigue, palpitations, muscle weakness, and general inability to cope could all be blamed on allergies.

Hill died in 2001, having seen her message become mainstream. But the rapid growth of allergy-fear has also prompted a growing number of skeptics to ask if the epidemic is not partly the latest bout of health hysteria that, in different incarnations, has hit the Western world from century to century. The skeptical science writer Caroline Richmond invented a spoof illness in the 1980s—allergy to bright clothes—and wrote to Hill warning her about it. Hill's organization publicized the illness, and before long, a small but growing group of people claimed they had it. When Hill was told it had been a joke, she insisted that bright clothes allergy really did exist, and thanked Richmond for having exposed it.

Other skeptics include Dr. Ephraim Kahn, the former chief of environmental epidemiology for Florida State Department of Health Services, who told the *San Francisco Chronicle,* "Most of the patients with this diagnosis are suffering from a variety of psychological and psychosomatic illnesses, particularly depression, which has a great deal of physical manifestations."

ALLERGIC TO REALITY?

Whether severe environmental allergies exist or not, many mild conditions seem to exist only in the minds of the sufferers and their doctors. An Ohio State University study of 246 students who were taking the prescription allergy drugs Claritin, Allegra, and Zyrtec, claims that 65 percent of the students were found not to have allergies when given blood tests.

The research presented in March 2001 to the American College of Osteopathic Family Physicians, proved controversial because it was funded by a blood-test manufacturer. But it is reinforced by a study by the British Nutrition Foundation which claims that while about 20 percent of the U.K. population believes it has a food allergy or intolerance, less than 3 percent of them actually do.

The Foundation's spokeswoman, Dr. Sarah Schenker, tells the London *Daily Telegraph* (November 5, 2001), "Quite wrongly, the 'reactions' have been blamed as the cause of weight gain and niggling health problems such as headaches, spots, upset digestion and general aches and pains. We are very concerned that people seem to be using food allergies and intolerance as an excuse for weight gain rather than cutting down on food and doing more exercise."

Car-Color Killers

Worried about road safety? You should be: around three thousand people are killed in crashes every day worldwide. And you are particularly at peril if the car in your garage is painted brown, black, or green.

But you could halve your chances of serious injury from an accident if your vehicle comes in a sensible shade of silver. Research conducted in New Zealand claims that drivers of silver cars face half the risk of a serious accident involving injury faced by other-car-color drivers.

Researcher Sue Furness of the University of Auckland says that brown, black, and green cars have the highest crash risk. Red, often considered the color of safety, is no better than blue, gray, yellow, or white, according to the report in the *British Medical Journal* (2003, 327; 7429:1455). The risk of a serious injury in yellow, gray, red, and blue cars is not so bad—and not significantly different from that in white cars.

Her research provoked a flurry of criticism about its methods, but it supports a study reported the previous year in *Epidemiology* (2002, 13; 6:721), which suggests that bright or light-colored vehicles such as yellow and white are safer, particularly on open roads in daylight, because they are more visible. The study used data from the Spanish database of traffic crashes from 1993 to 1999, which must have provided plenty to go on.

But Furness, who studied one thousand drivers in Auckland in 1998 and 1999, found silver to be safest color of all. She says, "Increasing the proportion of silver cars could be an effective strategy to reduce the burden of injury from car crashes." Why not go all the way and paint every car on the road silver? Of course, that might wreak havoc in the parking lot at the mall.

Legal Drug Drivers

On the other hand, you would still have to look out for elderly drivers so confused by their prescription drugs that they are unlikely to notice the existence of other traffic, let alone the color of your car.

Telling if an older person is too stoned on medication to drive is a difficult business. But one study of Canadian drivers from age sixty-seven to eighty-four found they were twice as likely to be in a serious car crash if they were on lithium to control their moods, reports the *British Medical Journal* (2004;

328:558–559). Other studies have found similar crash statistics involving some of the millions of elderly people prescribed benzodiazepine tranquilizers.

Christmas Crashers

Beyond drugs and paint colors, even family festivities can cause serious road accidents, claims Britain's Royal Automobile Club. The motoring organization's psychiatrists claim that car drivers are suffering "a deadly new syndrome"—festive auto disorder, or FAD, reports the London *Evening Standard* (December 23, 1997).

Symptoms, which strike during the season of good cheer, include extreme irritability and volatile disagreements among same-car occupants suffering a variety of "stress points" connected with Christmas and the mass migration toward family turkey dinners.

"Ill-feeling and simmering discontent between family members in the close confines of festive homes can boil over at the slightest provocation once they get behind the wheel," claims the psychologist Conrad King, who maintains that precisely 56 percent of in-car arguments are caused by bad map reading or getting lost. Backseat driving and unruly passengers are the next two most common causes of in-car family fallouts, he says.

"It is an important road-safety issue," King says. "The seasonal syndrome invariably involves arguments outside the car which eventually boil over in the confined space of the family sedan and cause distress on the road."

He adds: "People might also be aware of SAD [Seasonal Affective Disorder caused by lack of sunlight hitting the brain] and how that can lead to feeling down at this time of the year. But a combination of FAD and SAD could ruin anyone's Christmas."

cadillac arrests

You might be better off getting out of the car and walking. The air inside your vehicle can be more polluted than that outside—to the point where it damages your heart, warned the U.S. Environmental Protection Agency in May 2004.

The agency measured the pollution levels in nine police officers' squad cars and tested their blood levels for signs of harmful proteins that can lead to heart blockages. The levels were consistently higher at the end of their nine-hour patrol shifts than they had been at the start.

Robert Devlin, an agency researcher, says that even when you shut your car windows and close the air vents, there can be more harmful pollution inside your car than out on the street. Dangerous particles from your exhaust are sucked back inside and stay there in higher concentrations. The particles can be so small—one eight-hundredth the width of a human hair—that they pass through air filters.

Terminal airports

Fear of flying should not only affect people in the air. A ten-year study of two-hundred thousand people who live near Los Angeles International Airport warns how jet noise can propel you into an early grave.

Living near an airport can double your risk of killing

yourself, warn researchers in the German journal, *Schriften für Wasser Boden Lufthygiene* (1993; 88:428). Not only did suicides rise by more than 100 percent among people from age forty-five to fifty-four, but the number of accidental deaths jumped by 60 percent in older people. There was also a 5 percent increase in the number of deaths from disease, and nearly 18 percent more heart attacks. The researchers conclude that in areas around large airports, jet noise can cause an extra sixty deaths every year.

HEADACHE OR TUMOR?

What do you mean, it's not serious?

That ache, rash, pain, or occasional mystery symptom could well land you in the hospital—and things can go seriously downhill from there. Up to 13 percent of patients in hospitals and doctors' offices may in fact be suffering from simple hypochondria rather than a distinct physical illness, warns Oliver Howes, London Maudsley Hospital psychiatrist, in the *Lancet* (1998, 351; 9112:1332).

Unfortunately, hypochondriacs are frequently mistaken by busy doctors and nurses for people with real life-threatening illnesses. And this, ironically, causes a significant number of hypochondriacs to become ill by being sent for unnecessary medical investigations and operations, and given unnecessary and potentially harmful drugs. So before you dial the ambulance, think at least twice. . . .

Persistent Headache or Brain Cancer?

Risk rate: less than 1 percent
Something in the back of your mind tells you it's bound to be a tumor. In fact, this is extremely unlikely. Fewer than one in one hundred people with regular

headaches is found to develop a brain tumor. They are rare in people under age thirty and only about thirty-five hundred people develop one each year in England and Wales.

Still not convinced? These are the clinical signs: severe persistent headache; vomiting—sometimes suddenly; dizziness; fits; major seizures or local twitching; total loss of hearing or sense of smell; hallucinations; drowsiness; personality changes; or loss of coordination.

Otherwise, persistent headaches are more likely to be caused by inflamed sinuses, a misaligned jaw, migraine, tension, caffeine, and hangovers. Or of course, they could all be in the mind.

Absent-Mindedness or Alzheimer's?

Risk rate: 20 percent

So the memory's not what it used to be. Could be serious, though it might not be. Memory loss ranges in severity from simple absent-mindedness, through mild cognitive impairment, to full-blown whack-out dementias such as Alzheimer's.

Mild Cognitive Impairment

This is a mild form of memory loss with a long and forgettable name. People with this condition may have to work harder to remember things and they experience a more rapid rate of memory decline than their peers. If you develop it, you have a higher than average chance of getting Alzheimer's.

The youngest people Alzheimer's strikes are generally in their late fifties. There is no sure way to detect if you have it, other than seeing your doctor if symptoms get worrisome.

But there is the "aha!" test. If you temporarily forget a word, then get the feeling it is on the tip of your tongue, and finally recall it with a sense of "Aha! That's it," then your reactions seem healthy. This doesn't tend to happen with mild cognitive impairment and Alzheimer's.

Testicular Cancer Lump or Normal Plumbing?

Risk rate: 10 percent

Many cancer campaigners want men to rummage themselves monthly—or get a woman friend to check their balls for them. So after a bath or shower, while rolling the testicles between thumb and forefinger, you may find something troubling at the back of the scrotum. It's small, firm, and tubelike. Now breathe normally. It's the epididymis. It transports sperm. Only if you find other small lumps, irregularities, enlargements, or changes in firmness should you go to the doctor, just to be sure.

Floaters or Blindness?

Risk rate: 1 percent

The most common cause of disturbances in your field of vision are gray floaters—particles in the fluid at the back of the eye. People notice them more on bright days.

They shift as you glance around. It's normal to have one or two per eye. Hypochondriacs tend to notice them—and worry about them—much more. But if you do suddenly notice a large number, visit an ophthalmologist.

Flashing disturbances and double vision are a bit more worrisome. If they are accompanied by mind-blitzing headaches, then it sounds like migraine. They could be a result of your coming off benzodiazepine drugs, which are often prescribed for anxiety. They might be a symptom of high blood pressure, where visual disturbances can be accompanied by fatigue, breathlessness, ringing in the ears, and headaches.

And it might just—but only might just—indicate that a brain tumor is increasing the pressure in your skull.

HEART ATTACK OR HEARTBURN?

Risk rate: 5 percent

Shockingly painful burning sensation behind the breastbone? Acid taste in the throat? Just had a stressful lunch? Probably heartburn. Excess stomach acid heads up from the stomach, causing burning behind the breastbone and an acid taste in the throat. And yes, it can hurt a lot—gut juice is as corrosive as battery acid, and its production is boosted by stress.

The pain can be so severe that people think they are having a coronary. This can be ruled out with a simple ECG test. Are you already on first-name terms with the hospital ECG people? Take it as an early warning from your heart: being overweight and smoking makes heartburn worse, as well as massively increasing your chances of a coronary.

Palpitations or Heart Failure?

Risk rate: 2 percent

Heartbeat sometimes feels funny? Hypochondriacs are renowned for worrying about their heart rates. Practically everyone experiences some type of disturbed heartbeat now and then, but most don't go dashing to the doctor.

The palpitation is usually in the form of a mild flux or skipped beat. Your heart does not actually skip beats—the experience is called an ectopic heartbeat—you are really noticing a pulse that is not strong enough to be felt, followed by a relatively forceful beat.

People who fixate on their heart rate also fear that it is running too quickly, too slowly, or irregularly. Odd heart rates are called cardiac arrhythmias, though normally the arrhythmias are in the patient's head. A normal pulse is sixty to eighty beats a minute. Go on then, check it.

If you do have an irregular heartbeat, it could indicate that you will go on to develop more serious problems. Be worried if you have recurrent palpitations, chest discomfort, fainting, sweating, breathlessness, dizziness, or confusion.

If you are still worried, cut out recognized triggers such as coffee and alcohol. And stop worrying: the ancient poets were right—emotions do make hearts flutter, and the majority of ectopic heartbeats are due to emotional stress.

ALL IN THE MIND

But that doesn't mean it ain't lethal

CORROSIVE CHARACTERS

From the ancient Greeks to Shakespeare and beyond, the concept of tragedy has focused on the idea that people carry the seeds of their own destruction. This is reinforced by modern research which claims that your personality can predict the disease that will kill you.

Strange results from a study of Scottish people have prompted epidemiologists to claim that your temperament may be linked to the disease you ultimately die from. The researchers examined the records of 878 patients who died, out of a population of almost 10,000 Glasgow students. The students' temperaments had been recorded by a doctor over a twenty-year period from 1948–1968.

The report in the *Journal of Epidemiology and Community Health* (2003, 57; 11:888) says that nearly one in ten of the original group had been found to have an "unstable" temperament. Those who had been diagnosed as having manic depression, more fashionably called bipolar disorder, had a higher risk of dying of a heart attack. Those who had been diagnosed as being abnormally anxious were more likely to have died of cancer.

Anxiety Attacks

Further evidence that you can fret yourself to death comes from a Norwegian study of more than sixty thousand people, which again suggests that people prone to anxiety are more likely to get cancer. The eight-year survey by psychiatrists at the University of Bergen, reported in *New Scientist* (May 31, 2003), found that people who score highly in anxiety tests are 25 percent more likely to develop either cancers or abnormal cells.

From Fretful to Forgetful

More reasons to worry: scientists studying Alzheimer's disease say they have discovered data which indicates that people who are prone to feeling distressed are more likely to develop dementia.

Researchers in Chicago analyzed the results of a study of 797 people in religious orders who, at the average age of seventy-five, were Alzheimer's-free. They were given neurological examinations and measured for their ability to worry about things on a "Neuroticism Scale."

In the following five years, 140 of the people studied started to suffer dementia. The medical researchers report in *Neurology* (2003, 61; 11:1479) that for every point higher up the Neuroticism Scale a person scored, his or her risk of Alzheimer's increased by 6 percent. Being an intensive worrier can double your risk of the disease, they conclude.

But why? Dr. Robert Wilson, of the Rush-Presbyterian-St. Luke's Medical Center in Chicago, claims that long-term stress seems to create changes in the brain's hippocampus, which plays a role in memory function. Does that mean that giving people stress-busting antidepressants will cut people's risk of Alzheimer's? The doctors say they don't know.

Denture Dementia

Perhaps your Alzheimer's risk has more to do with your teeth. Researchers writing in the *Psychiatric Bulletin* (1992; 16:227) checked 159 patients with Alzheimer's and found that half of them wore dentures—a much larger proportion than is normal for people their age.

The researchers, from the London Institute of Psychiatry, also found an increased level of family history of dementia in patients with false teeth, which they say "suggests a genetic predisposition towards both." But the link may have more to do with jaws than genes.

The lead researcher, Alistair Burns, and his team also found, using brain scans, an association between false teeth and brain cells dying in the temporal lobe. This "may be the result of reduced chewing, leading to a disuse atrophy of the limbic system," he reports.

Seasonal Schizophrenia

Chewing each mouthful of food forty-two times might help to stave off Alzheimer's, but your risk of developing another common form of mental illness may come down to something as simple as your birthday.

Being born at the wrong time of year can increase your chance of developing schizophrenia, claims Dr. J. M. Eagles, who studied more than thirty-five hundred people diagnosed as schizophrenic born between 1900 and 1969. His article, in the *British Journal of Psychiatry* (1995, 167; 4:469), reports that men born in the winter or spring months are significantly more likely to develop the disorder than men born in the rest of the year.

That correlation is getting stronger as the years go by, for reasons Dr. Eagles cannot explain. He adds, however, that for women, the birthday/schizophrenia link is weak, and growing steadily weaker.

Birthday Blues

For women, birthdays are not only bad news if they hate the idea of being yet another year older. Women are more likely to die in the week after their birthday than any other week in the year, says a study of more than 2 million people's deaths, published in *Psychosomatic Medicine* (1992, 54; 5:532).

Why? This phenomenon shows that many women really do in fact look forward to their birthdays. Female death rates dip in the weeks beforehand, which indicates that women are hanging on for all the birthday cards and the presents, say sociologists at the University of California, San Diego. The death rate then leaps in the following week. So there's no point buying them any long books as a present.

Festive Fatalities

Failing to enjoy big cultural celebrations could mean missing out on months of life. People who consider such events important may live longer, according to a study of the mortality rates of people in religious groups around significant annual festivals.

A survey of Jewish people found that their death rates fell sharply below the expected level before Passover and rose by an equal amount above the expected level shortly afterward. The University of California study in the *Lancet* (1988, 2; 8613:728) reports that, in contrast, non-Jewish control groups showed no significant fluctuation in mortality rates around Passover. The pattern is most pronounced in the years when Passover falls on a weekend, when it is most likely to be celebrated by the largest number of people, say the researchers.

The same team reported a similar effect two years later among Chinese people around the date of the Harvest Moon Festival which, like Passover and other major cultural and religious ceremonies, involves an annual family get-together with lots of food. The researchers found that deaths fall by a third in the weeks before the festival, and rise by a compensatory third in the weeks afterward. The biggest dip in deaths is from strokes, followed by heart attacks and tumors.

On the Other Hand . . .

Big public holidays can prove such a miserable disappointment that the risk of suicides takes a big leap shortly afterward, warns a report in *Suicide and Life Threatening Behaviour* (1999, 29; 3:272). Danish researchers call this the "broken-promise effect" and say that their study of thirty-two thousand of their compatriots over twenty-five years shows that an increase in suicides is particularly noticeable just after the major public holidays of Christmas, Easter, and Whitsunday.

Friday the 13th Phenomenon

If you believe certain dates can signify ill omens, then they really might prove unfortunate, says a study that found an unusually high number of Japanese and Chinese people suffer heart deaths on "bad luck" days.

Researchers at California University, San Diego, noted that the number four is considered a bad omen in Japanese and Chinese cultures, particularly because it is close in sound to "death" in some Southeast Asian languages. So they examined mortality rates on the fourth day of each month, and discovered that these are the peak days for Japanese and Chinese cardiac fatalities in hospitals.

They compared this phenomenon with death rates among white Americans—for whom the fourth of each month is just an ordinary day (with the exception, of course, of the fourth of July). The scientists report in the *British Medical Journal* (2001; 323(7327):1443) that for white America it is statistically just like any other heart-death day.

The researchers have christened the phenomenon the *Hound of the Baskervilles Effect,* after the fatally frightening dog from the Sherlock Holmes book.

The peak-death effect on the fourth of the month was not followed by a compensatory dip in heart deaths on subsequent days among Japanese and Chinese patients. So the effect might not simply hit people who were going to have a heart attack anyway. It may prey on those who

would never have died around that time—
had they not been scared to death by
superstition.

BLUE-LIPPED MONDAY

In many industrialized societies, miserable Monday
mornings are a lethal problem, according to research
from Germany and Italy, which shows that heart attacks
are most common as the week begins. Experts blame it
on the stress of returning to work after the weekend.

The six-year study of more than twenty-six hundred
Germans, coordinated by researchers at the Free University of Berlin, showed that the average person has a 20
percent higher chance of having a heart attack on a Monday than on any other day. The report, in *Circulation*
(1994, 90; 1:87), reveals that work is to blame: employed
Germans have a 33 percent higher death risk at the start
of the week. Nonworkers, by comparison, have no increase in risk.

Meanwhile, a study in the *European Heart Journal*
(1994, 15; 7:882) of eleven thousand Italians by the
Luigi Sacco Hospital in Milan has identified 8 AM on a
Monday morning as the most stressful time for the heart.
Both the German and Italian studies showed that Sunday
is the least stressful point of the week for working men.

Weekend Woe

Monday is not the worst day for everyone, though.
While Japanese men's heart-fatality rates increase by a

quarter on Mondays, Japanese women's cardiac death rates jump by more than a third on Saturdays, say Osaka University doctors. They admit in *Heart* (2003, 89; 4:398) that they are not certain of the women's precise risk factors but speculate that Saturdays signal the start of "a stressful weekend burden for women." Yes, hubby's home.

Death by Grieving

You really can die from a broken heart, claim studies of bereaved people. That may seem understandable enough, but then it gets weird—the survey results show that the very manner in which a loved one dies can determine the type of illness that threatens the people who mourn the deceased.

A large-scale study of fifteen thousand bereaved men and women in Israel says it has found that women are 50 percent more likely to die in the first six months after losing their partner. The rate of increase in men is 40 percent.

Inexplicably, the lethal impact of bereavement is greater on more educated men, say the researchers from Jerusalem's Hebrew University School of Public Health and Community Medicine in *Social Science Medicine* (2003, 56; 2:405).

The hand-from-the-grave effect has a powerful influence in determining what illnesses bereaved people will suffer, claim Dutch researchers in *Family Practitioner* (1988, 5; 4:278). Their study of 313 bereaved people found that they are more likely to suffer a minor illness if their loved one died after a chronic illness. Bereaved people are more likely to suffer a serious illness if they have been confronted with the sudden death of a loved one, say the Dutch scientists, from the Nijmegen University Department of General Practice.

A study of 95,647 widowed Finns claims that in the first fortnight after losing a spouse, your risk of dying of a heart attack doubles. And in the month after a partner dies, your chances of dying in a violent incident such as an accident are doubled, the researchers write in the *American Journal of Public Health* (1987, 77; 3: 283).

Twin Trouble

While the death of a partner increases your chances of dying in the following twelve months, having your twin die increases your chances of following suit in the second subsequent year, warn scientists at King's College, London.

Their study of Danish deaths shows the effect is stronger for identical twins— and can shorten the lives of both men and women in a similar manner, they report in *Twin Research* (2002, 5; 3:210).

Culture Crazy

Is your nationality driving you mad? The American Psychiatric Association's 1997 *Diagnostic and Statistical Manual of Mental Disorders,* known by professionals as DSM-IV, lists strange syndromes peculiar to particular cultures. As any globe-trotter worth his tattered backpack knows, all the world's nations are mad. They just happen to fall victim to different local madnesses.

The diagnostic manual points out that if you are Malaysian, you may rush into the clinic suffering from *koro,* a mental illness where the sufferer is gripped by the belief that intense anxiety will make his penis (or her vulva and nipples) recede into the body and possibly cause death.

Inuit or Eskimo? *Pibloktoq* could be a problem. It's a sort of snow rage. "During the attack, the individual may tear off his or her clothing, break furniture, shout obscenities, eat feces, flee from protective shelters, or perform other irrational or dangerous acts," says the manual.

As a Japanese person, you may develop *taijin kyofusho,* which can manifest itself as a dread of embarrassment.

Indian men can suffer from *jiryan.* The main symptoms are feelings of weakness and worry associated with the discharge of semen.

Chinese male? There is always the danger of *shen-k'uei,* a "life-threatening" loss of semen leaking out in urine, again caused by anxiety. You could try relaxing with some gentle exercise, but that could spark *Qi-gong psychotic reaction,* characterized by acute paranoid symptoms after overindulging in qi-gong, a system of exercises that forms the basis of t'ai chi.

If you are South American, a bout of *susto*—soul loss caused by a frightening experience—might be in the cards. Or you may be in line for an *ataque de nervios,* a brief outburst of dramatic, disturbed behavior following an emotional shock.

And if you hail from the Middle East, you could contract *zar.* Symptoms include shouting, laughing, hitting your head against a wall, singing, or weeping, then sinking into apathetic withdrawal because you believe you are possessed by spirits. That would get you heavily sedated in the West, but "such behavior is not considered pathological locally," says the manual.

The British doctors' newspaper, *Pulse* (June 3, 2002), adds some more definitions for worldwide weirdness. *Brain fag,* for example, is found in Nigerian and other African students. It is distinct from academic stress, and features burning or crawling sensations under the skin, visual disturbances, fatigue, and disrupted concentration. *Studiation madness* is a term used in Trinidad for a similar syndrome.

Latah, meanwhile, mainly affects Southeast Asians and North Eurasians. Victims mimick people's posture and voices, and erupt into obscene yells when startled. An apparently identical syndrome in Siberia is called *myriachit.* In Lappland it is called *Lapp panic.*

Westerners might think we can laugh smugly at all of this. But not so fast, says *Pulse* author Dr. Stefan Cembrowicz. Intentional drug overdoses are very rare in some cultures, for instance, among Africans in the Caribbean, but they are extremely common in Europe and America. Likewise with anorexia. Perhaps these are also culturally bound syndromes, he suggests.

Fishy Odor Fear

That funny smell? Is it you? If you are a woman, you are more likely to think you smell funny, according to researchers at St. Mary's Hospital Medical School, London, in the *Lancet* (1995, 345; 869:1308). In response to a newspaper article about strange bodily odors, the scientists were contacted by 187 members of the public who thought they smelled rotten. Most felt they smelled of fish. Others feared they had a cheesy odor, and a few believed they had a strong tang of rotten food.

When the word spread, more than seven times more women than men got in touch, saying they smelled anything from fishy to "vaguely unpleasant." When questioned, however, they said they were the only person to notice it—family, friends, and colleagues thought nothing was amiss.

The researchers christened the problem *body malodor syndrome* and suggest that these people may suffer from cacosmia, a condition where people apparently perceive perfectly innocuous odors as offensive.

COLLECT THESE SYNDROMES

A syndrome is defined as a range of apparently unlinked symptoms in a patient that some sharp-eyed medic notices all share the same underlying cause. In ancient Greek, *syn drom* means to run together. Ambitious researchers know that if you can convincingly nail several symptoms together and blame them on a zeitgeisty cause, then bingo, you have carved your name in the annals of medical history—and given us all something new to worry about.

Media Malaise

Be on your guard against *information fatigue syndrome* (IFS), apparently caused by being bombarded with business data and mass media. Sufferers feel compelled to search constantly for more information. They experience anxiety and sleeplessness, as well as increasing doubt about their decision-making abilities.

Psychologist Dr. David Lewis warned the world of IFS in a Reuters report, *Dying for Information,* in 1996. He says the syndrome is a direct result of the information revolution, and adds that having too much information can be as dangerous as having too little. His report interviewed business executives and concluded that 52 percent suffered from it.

The illness rapidly developed its own instant victims and mythology. London's *Daily Telegraph* on October 12, 1996, interviewed an IFS sufferer about her painful five-year recovery. On April 20 the following year, Edward Welsh reported in the *Sunday Times* that the syndrome had first been detected in American intelligence officers in the Second World War.

Historic Histrionics

There is real history afoot with *Stendhal's syndrome,* which strikes culture vultures gazing at Florence's Renaissance treasures. Italian doctors warn that trying to see too many artistic and historical artifacts in too short a time can cause dizziness, panic, paranoia, and even madness.

It is called Stendhal's syndrome because the nineteenth-century French novelist is said to have been the first to write about the head-spinning disorientation some tourists experience when they encounter Florentine masterpieces. When Stendhal saw Giotto's ceiling frescoes at Santa Croce, he was overcome. "Life was drained from me. I walked with the fear of falling," he wrote in 1817.

But Stendhal was not the only day-tripper to go all dizzy. In the late 1970s, Dr. Graziella Magherinie, the head of psychiatry at Florence's Santa Maria Nuova Hospital, noticed that many of the tourists who visited Florence were overcome with anything from temporary panic attacks to bouts of psychosis lasting several days. She named the temporary amnesia and disorientation Stendhal's syndrome.

You are most likely to be struck down by it if you are

- Ages twenty-six to forty
- Sensitive and impressionable
- A lone traveler visiting a gallery on a whim
- Sightseeing without a professional guide.

Note, too, *Jerusalem syndrome,* which was identified in 1987 and is said to afflict tourists who feel oddly compelled to visit the Holy City and are overcome by encountering its ancient sites. In February 2004, Nathan Coley, a visual artist, was awarded £10,000 to investigate why between five and ten people a year find themselves clinically intoxicated by the Holy City.

Banging Heads

Even at home, your brain could go bang. In 1890, the phenomenon was described as a "bolt driven through the head." A 1920 report said it was "as if something had snapped or given way in my brain." *Exploding head syndrome* (EHS) is probably quite common, but what causes it, says Dr. Howard Seiden in the *Toronto Star* (March 29, 1990) remains a medical mystery.

The main symptom is noise like an explosion, accompanied by fear or terror and sometimes a sudden flash of light. It generally occurs during sleep, while a person is dropping off, and less commonly while waking. Sufferers are mainly middle-aged or older and it is more common in women than men.

FAKE FAMILY FEAR

Do you ever get the feeling you are surrounded by phonies? In 1923, a fifty-three-year-old French woman complained that her family had been replaced by identical doubles. Later, she began to feel the same about friends and neighbors, and eventually feared that even she herself was being shadowed by a double. It was the first recorded case of *Capgras's syndrome,* which appears to result from damage to a "sense of familiarity" pathway within the brain.

Since then about three hundred others have been diagnosed with the syndrome. Capgras patients typically believe they live in a world of impersonators. The feeling is strongest among close family and friends but can extend to pets and places. Some years ago, a man in England was so sure his father had been replaced by a robot that he slashed his throat open, trying to find the wires.

Researchers believe Capgras's syndrome is caused by a failure of normal recognition processes following brain damage from a stroke, drug overdose, or some other cause. Sufferers can still recognize people and places, but no longer get the physiological buzz of familiarity that normally goes with such recognition.

Sightless Seers

Perhaps you are blind, but don't know it. Sightless people with *Anton's syndrome* deny that they are blind. This seems to happen when two different areas of the brain have been damaged: the one needed for seeing and the one needed for knowing that you are seeing. It occurs quite suddenly, often after a stroke, and victims of Anton's syndrome may walk around for quite some time bumping into things and having other mishaps until they become convinced something is wrong.

Anarchist's Arm

Or maybe your body is about to rebel on you. In *anarchic hand syndrome,* first recognized in 1908, sufferers lose control of one hand—which acts of its own free will, causing frustration and embarrassment in equal measures. It is also known as the *Dr. Strangelove syndrome,* after the 1963 film, *Dr. Strangelove,* in which Peter Sellers had to fight vigorously with his arm to stop it from making Nazi salutes.

It is believed to be caused by damage to an area deep in the central brain, near the forehead, as a result of viruses, head injuries, or strokes. There is no known cure. A case was sent to the Dutch courts after a man claiming to have the syndrome was arrested for pinching the bottom of an airline stewardess on a KLM flight. Another poor victim is reported to have been unable to stop his hand from masturbating him in public, says a report in the *American Journal of Physical Medicine and Rehabilitation* (2000, 79; 4:395).

Foreign Accent Syndrome

So you wake up one day to find you can't help talking with a foreign accent. That will be the rare, and apparently neurological, disorder called *foreign accent syndrome.* In November 2003, Professor Jack Ryalis, a speech expert at the University of Central Florida, reported how a local woman, Tiffany Noell, recovered from a stroke to find herself speaking with a British accent. She had never been to the United Kingdom, her family and friends found it hard to understand her, and locals kept asking where she came from. She became agoraphobic and refused to go out.

When Ryalis diagnosed her, she no longer felt mad and decided to make the condition more widely recognized and understood. Things could have been worse for Noell. There have only been about twenty cases, and one of the earliest known involved a Norwegian woman recovering from shrapnel injuries following the German invasion of Norway. She developed what sounded like a strong German accent and was ostracized by her community.

Cases of foreign accent syndrome have different causes and results, which can, for example, make a native English speaker sound Spanish or Dutch. The accent a patient develops is not dependent on any knowledge of a particular foreign language. It is rather the combination of certain changed features, such as lengthening of syllables, altered pitch, or mispronounced sounds, which make a patient's pronunciation sound foreign.

Other cases include an English speaker from Massachusetts who walked away from a car accident speaking with a French accent. Oxford neuropsychologists have recently located some very small lesions in the victim's brain that they claim to be the cause.

And on the Third Stroke . . .

You might have developed *horologagnosia,* a complete inability to tell time. Dr. Luke Kartsounis, of the National Hospital for Neurology and Neuro-surgery in London, discovered the condition when treating a fifty-seven-year-old man who had just had a right-sided stroke.

Stroke victims often have difficulty making sense of visual information, but Dr. Kartsounis reported the case in the *Journal of Neurology, Neuroscience, and Psychiatry* (1990, 30; 4:647). While the sufferer scored well in language and memory tests, and could see the hands, the face, and the numbers on the clock, he could no longer tell time.

"If you asked him to set the hands on the clockface at a particular time, he had no problem. But he could not read what he was doing," says Dr. Kartsounis. "He would say: the small hand is on eight, and the large hand is on twelve. If you asked him what time it was, he might give— on repeated prompting—a silly answer, like eight minutes to twelve."

Fortunately, the victim started to recover after a few weeks, and became rather more clock-wise.

cartoon crazy

Mysterious lesions in the brain can plunge you into a strange cartoonlike fantasy world, if you suddenly develop *Lhermitte's peduncular hallucinosis.*

In 1922, the French neurologist Jean Lhermitte treated a seventy-two-year-old woman who experienced bizarre visual hallucinations involving strange-looking chickens, people attired in odd costumes, and children playing. Although the patient knew the hallucinations were not real, she would sometimes try to touch them. When she died, Lhermitte discovered the probable cause: a lesion in her midbrain.

The case was described by neurologists Anthony Risser and Frank Powell at the 45th Annual Meeting of the American Academy of Neurology in New York in April 1993. They also reported cases of a female patient who repeatedly saw the head of a dog or an image of an animal's body projected on to a wall in her home; a male sufferer who witnessed pictures of his grandmother flashed on the wall, as if projected in a home movie; and a man who used to watch a toy monster moving around, "being vivid, colorful, and non-threatening."

Other patients had visions of lions jumping into the room through a window, silver and golden fish swimming below the bed, and Asian people walking in a single line down a hallway with their hands grasped together in prayer.

The worst thing, it seems, about developing Lhermitte's peduncular hallucinosis is having to pronounce the name of your disorder. Almost everyone who has had the condition reportedly found it rather entertaining.

57 Varieties of Fear

You can, it seems, get phobic about pretty much anything. Some people are scared of otters. Others live in
fear of amputees. And some folk are frightened by knees.
Have fun with fear—create your own new phobia.
These fifty-seven have already been done.

Ablutophobia   Fear of washing
Alektorophobia   Fear of chickens
Allodoxaphobia   Fear of opinions
Anginophobia   Fear of sore throats
Anthophobia   Fear of flowers
Apotemnophobia   Fear of amputees
Arachibutyrophobia   Fear of peanut butter
Automatonophobia   Fear of ventriloquists' dummies
Bibliophobia   Fear of books
Bogyphobia   Fear of demons and goblins
Cacophobia   Fear of ugliness
Caligynephobia or venustraphobia   Fear of beau-
   tiful women
Cathisophobia or kathisophobia   Fear of sitting
   down
Chinophobia   Fear of snow
Chorophobia   Fear of dancing
Coitophobia or genophobia   Fear of having sexual
   intercourse
Cyberphobia or logizomechanophobia   Fear of
   computers
Enosiophobia or enissophobia   Fear of having
   committed an unpardonable sin
Eosophobia   Fear of dawn or daylight
Euphobia   Fear of hearing good news

Geniophobia   Fear of chins
Genuphobia   Fear of knees
Graphophobia   Fear of writing or handwriting
Hobophobia   Fear of beggars
Homilophobia   Fear of sermons
Hygrophobia   Fear of liquids, dampness, or moisture
Kosmikophobia   Fear of cosmic phenomena
Lacanophobia   Fear of vegetables
Listophobia   Fear of lists
Liticaphobia   Fear of lawsuits
Lutraphobia   Fear of otters
Macrophobia   Fear of long waits
Melophobia   Fear or hatred of music
Metrophobia   Fear or hatred of poetry
Mnemophobia   Fear of memories
Myrmecophobia   Fear of ants
Nomatophobia   Fear of names
Novercaphobia or pentheraphobia   Fear of mothers-in-law
Octophobia   Fear of the number eight
Panophobia or panphobia or pantaphobia   Fear of everything
Peladophobia   Fear of bald people
Phobophobia   Fear of fear
Pluviophobia   Fear of being rained on
Politicophobia   Fear of politicians
Proctophobia or rectophobia   Fear of the rectum or rectal diseases
Pteronophobia   Fear of being tickled by feathers
Sesquipedalophobia   Fear of long words
Teratophobia   Fear of giving birth to monsters
Tremophobia   Fear of trembling
Venerophobia   Fear of venereal disease
Vestiphobia   Fear of clothing

Wiccaphobia   Fear of witches and witchcraft
Xanthophobia   Fear of color yellow or word yellow
Xerophobia   Fear of dryness
Xylophobia   Fear of wooden objects
Zeusophobia   Fear of God or gods
Zoophobia   Fear of animals

Death Is Contagious

Celebrity suicides could increase your chance of ending it all—depending on where you learn about them first. A study in *Injury Prevention* (2002, 8; 4:IV30) found that when high-profile political or showbiz personalities kill themselves and become newspaper stories, there is a dramatic increase in the number of copycat suicides.

Televised stories about such people do not have the same effect, nor do plotlines about soap-opera characters, claims the researchers at a Detroit university.

Copycat Crashes

Suicide has a bad effect on people's motoring safety, according to a study in the journal *Science* (1977; 196:1464), which seems to suggest that the best thing to do in your car is switch off the radio news and listen to something cheerful. The researchers found that motor vehicle deaths increase just after suicide stories are broadcast on the media.

Knockout Knock-on

Even if you are in a cheerful mood, if you look like a failed prizefighter you should watch out after high-profile boxing matches. A study in the *American Sociology Review* (1983; 48:560) shows that murder rates go up after televised fights where there is lots of money offered to the winner, and that your chances of being murdered post-fight rise sharply if you bear a physical resemblance to the losing boxer. The greater the amount of publicity given to the story, the higher the subsequent rise in deaths.

BAD STARTS TO LIFE

And from then on, it's all downhill

HAPPY CHILDHOOD? ROTTEN LUCK

Psychologists who followed the lives of 1,216 children assessed in 1922 found that those who were rated as more cheerful and optimistic, and as having a strong sense of humor, died earlier in adult life than those who were less cheerful.

The research flies in the face of the new trend for "positive psychology," which focuses on boosting happiness rather than alleviating misery as a way of improving your health. Positive psychology is based on findings such as a Yale University psychologists' study of 660 volunteers ages fifty and older, which found that thinking positively about aging may add an average of seven-and-a-half years to your life. The team, led by Dr. Becca Levy, suggests in the *Journal of Personality and Social Psychology* (2002, 83; 2:261) that having an optimistic attitude can bolster the will to live, although they admit they can't explain it fully.

But that would not impress the cheerful-child researchers from the University of California, the State University of New York Medical School, and La Sierra University Riverside, California. They say that the happy youngsters they followed "grew up to be more likely to

die in any given year but not more likely to die
of any particular cause."

The researchers found that the cheerful kids
grew up more likely to drink, smoke, and take
more risks—possibly because their optimism makes the
dangers appear smaller to them. But still the scientists
add: "These behaviors cannot fully explain their relatively early deaths."

The report, in *Personality and Social Psychology Bulletin* (2002; 28:1155), concludes, "Although optimism
and positive emotions have been shown to have positive
effects when people are faced with short-term crisis, the
long-term effects of cheerfulness are more complex and
seem not entirely positive."

War? Brutality? Blame the Parents

Blame your upbringing for your controlling, tyranni-
cal tendencies. Were it not for bad parenting, the world
could have been spared dictators such as Saddam Hussein, Hitler, Stalin, and Idi Amin, according to American
war psychologist Jerome Frank.

Frank, an emeritus professor of psychiatry at Johns
Hopkins Medical School, argues that the modern age's
worst tyrants shared "strikingly similar" brutal formative
years. He writes in *Medicine and War* (March 1994) that
Hussein's early childhood was dominated by a brutal
stepfather who raised him in abject squalor. As a child,
Hussein displayed typical symptoms of early abuse, being
"angry, suspicious, guarded and self-centered."

His mother was remarkably aggressive. She once reportedly screamed at a doctor, "You son of a bitch, if my

daughter dies I will erect your gallows outside the hospital and hang you." The doctor fainted.

The Stalins were also unpopular neighbors, writes Frank. Joseph Stalin's father, a violent drunk who often subjected him to savage and undeserved beatings, died in a barroom brawl. His mother also thrashed him regularly. Frank says that as an adult, Stalin became preoccupied with beatings as a way of securing confessions. He was also noted for his unfailing memory for insult and injury.

The families of the deposed Ugandan dictator, Idi Amin, and Adolf Hitler also merited the intervention of social services, the professor says. Amin's parents split before he was born, and he may never have known his father. While he was a child, his mother slept with passing soldiers and practiced witchcraft.

Then there was Hitler, whose upbringing featured a self-perpetuating cycle of violence. His remote, authoritarian father was a harsh disciplinarian who was himself brutalized in childhood.

Professor Frank, also the author of *Sanity and Survival in the Nuclear Age,* says all four leaders grew up believing violence to be an appropriate means of resolving arguments, and may have developed extreme bloodthirstiness as a way of coping with the "death anxiety" instilled by their childhood terrors. Poor lambs.

Prenatal Delinquents

Another reason to blame your mother: pregnant women who smoke are four times more likely to have delinquent sons, claim Chicago University researchers. They say their study of 177 children shows that moms who smoke more than ten cigarettes a day put their boys at far greater risk of *conduct disorder*—the modern clinical term for lying, bullying, thieving, and vandalism.

Maternal smoking may inhibit development in the unborn baby's brain so it is less able to produce the feel-good drug, serotonin, and this may lead to thrill-seeking behaviors, suggest the child-development experts in the American Medical Association's *Archives of General Psychiatry* (1997, 54; 7:670).

On the other hand, psychologists at the University of Illinois at Chicago say the link could come down to good old-fashioned heredity. They report in *Addictive Behaviors* (2004, 29; 2:273) that mothers who smoke during pregnancy are markedly more likely to have been delinquents themselves. Like mother, like son.

Is Your Dread Fate in Your Palm?

Palmistry might seem a load of fairground nonsense, but our fingerprints and palms do seem to be accurate predictors of future health fortunes, argue researchers in the *British Medical Journal* (1993, 307; 6901:405).

Their study followed 139 babies born around fifty years ago in Lancashire, England, whose birth weight, placental weight, head circumference, and length at birth were recorded. Then they looked at the subjects' fingerprints and palmprints to see if they had any whorls—patterns formed when the lines on the fingerprints go beyond the usual arches or loops and become complete circles.

The ninety-three men and women with a whorl pattern on one or more fingers had significantly higher blood pressure than the forty-six people who did not have whorls.

The researchers believe this is because people who are thin at birth are apparently more likely to have whorls on their hands. They also have a higher risk of blood-pressure problems, possibly due to fetal undernutrition. Fingerprint patterns are, the researchers say, accurate markers for patterns for fetal growth—rather like rings in trees.

No, No—It's Your Ear

That fleshy protuberance on the left side of your head could hold vital clues to your chances of a heart attack. Doctors examining cadavers have noticed over the years that people killed by cardiac trouble seem much more likely to have a diagonal crease on their left ear lobe.

Researchers at St. Thomas's Hospital, London, specu-lated in the 1980s that the left ear is linked with the heart when a fetus is growing in the womb, and may show re-lated abnormalities by having a crease after birth.

America's Dr. Robert Superko goes further in his 2004 book, *Before the Heart Attacks,* claiming you need to look for a forty-five-degree diagonal crease on both ears. The cofounder of California's Berkeley HeartLab says the crease points upward toward your eyebrows, and sug-gests, "since both heart disease and ear creases are inher-ited, we think that these genes are somehow bundled together . . . this ear crease does act as an informal pre-dictive marker for increased risk."

Not everyone is convinced. The textbook, *Cardiac Diseases,* published by Harcourt International, says the association may be flawed because people get more ear creases the older they get.

Hairy ears could be a bad omen, though. The Harcourt authors add that the presence of hair in the ear canal has also been linked with increased risk of coronary disease.

Life Gives You the Finger

Now look at your hand again. Scientists at England's Liverpool University claim that the ratio of finger length to body height can indicate if a man is liable to suffer depression.

Their study of 102 men and women in *Evolution and Human Behaviour* (1999; 20:203) concludes that the longer a man's fingers are relative to his height, the more likely he is to get the blues. The strongest single indicator is the relative length of his wedding ring finger.

The study suggests that low levels of prenatal testosterone, produced from the eighth week of pregnancy, rather than day-by-day testosterone levels in adults is responsible. Dr. John Manning of the Liverpool University School of Biological Sciences says, "Men who experienced high concentrations of foetal testosterone have relatively long fingers—in particular, fourth digits which are longer than their second digits." So ladies, if you're checking to see if he's married, get a glimpse into how happy his (and your) future might be.

Pinkie Paternity

This is not the first time Dr. Manning has identified a hidden significance in finger length. In 1998 he established a link between the relative length of women's ring fingers and their fertility levels: women with ring fingers shorter than their forefingers tend to have high fertility. Conversely, men with relatively long ring fingers are more likely to have high fertility.

Ratio Rage

Being asymmetrical could lead you into violent confrontations, warn psychologists who claim that having different-sized ears, feet, wrists, hands, and ankles can severely affect your life chances.

Ohio State University researchers tried to provoke one hundred men and women around age twenty by asking them to solicit charity donations over the phone. The study subjects did not know that the people at the other end of the line were scripted to answer them confrontationally. The psychologists say in the *American Journal of Human Biology* (2004, 16; 4:458) that they measured how hard each of the study subjects slammed the receiver down after being rebuffed, and found that those who had the least physical symmetry were most likely to respond aggressively to provocation.

This won't only lead people into barroom brawls, says the researchers' leader, Dr. Zeynep Benderlioglu. He says being asymmetrical is a sign that you were born after an "environmentally challenged" pregnancy. In an earlier report in the same journal (2004, 16; 3:298) he studied

205 men and women and found that people born in winter and spring had a much higher chance of having badly matched ears and hands. He claims that people born in these seasons tend to live less long, and says this may explain it.

Winter-Birth Woe

More seasonal strangeness comes from American researchers led by the National Cancer Institute who say that your risk of developing a brain tumor is highest if you were born in January or February—and lowest if your birthday is in July or August.

In their study of 1,485 people, the increased risk was particularly noticeable in people who are either left-handed or ambidextrous, they write in *Neurology* (2004; 63:276). But why? The researchers aren't sure, but they also suggest that there may be something seasonal in the environment that is to blame.

SHORT-CHANGED

Here's something else to worry about that you can't alter—your height. You are apparently cursed for life if you grow slowly in the first twelve months after birth. This will affect your blood pressure—and it will also lower your income, believes a researcher at Southampton University in Great Britain.

Professor David Barker says his results hold true regardless of family or class, and that this suggests that slow infant growth may be accompanied by impaired brain development. The researcher revealed his findings at the Second World Congress on the Fetal Origins of Adult Disease, saying, "biological processes linked to poor growth in infancy lead to lifelong impairment of cognitive function with consequent lower occupational status and income." In layman's terms, it means being short is likely to leave you dumb, low-rent, and poor.

Dr. Barker, the author of *The Best Start in Life,* has pioneered research into how adult diseases begin in the womb, based on a study of 4,630 men born in Helsinki between 1934 and 1944. Research from his group has also shown that low infant growth is also linked to a later risk of death from heart disease and type 2 diabetes, as well as less impressive bank accounts.

"Although children who are short at any age up to puberty tend to do less well educationally and have lower incomes in later life, most of the action is in the first year," he says. "There are two organs that are not complete when the baby's born—one of them is the brain. And brain development between birth and one is known to be important. The liver is also not complete, and the liver sets how the body handles cholesterol, which is probably the link with heart disease.

"Weight at one year in boys predicts their cognitive function. Boys who grow better between birth and one have better educational achievements and they make more money when they're 50," he says. "Since, in a democratic society, income is a test of cognitive function among other things, this is rather a striking demonstration of the critical period of growth between birth and one year."

Speak upward

Being afflicted by small babyhood is also behind Swedish doctors' claim that short people are more likely to go deaf in old age. Their study of 479 men, reported in the *British Medical Journal* (2002, 327; 7425:1199), led them to conclude that age-related disorders such as hearing loss happen earlier if you are born with low levels of human growth hormone.

Proportional Problems

It is not only lack of height that can cause trouble. Proportions can also play a part, say Australian investigators, who have found that women whose legs are short compared with the rest of their bodies are at greater risk of developing type 2 diabetes. They report in *Diabetes Care* (2004; 27:1033) how they compared 222 women's statures and found that the ones with diabetes were on average 2.8 cm shorter—but they were not smaller all over: the difference in height was due entirely to their leg lengths, which were on average 3.2 cm shorter.

On the Other Hand . . .

Being tall can kill. A Bristol University study in the *Journal of Epidemiology and Community Health* (2000, 54; 2:97) warns that lankiness is associated with an increased risk of dying from some cancers, particularly blood, colon, and rectal cancers and, for men, prostate cancer.

And tall men are more likely than shorties to commit suicide, an American university study found. Men shorter than five feet six inches are particularly less prone to self-destruct, says the sociologist Dr. Steven Stack in the *Journal of Social Psychology* (1996, 136; 2:255). He suggests this is because diminutive men have to develop better psychological self-defense skills when young to compensate for their lack of stature and the bullies it attracts.

Being really tall is apparently the worst health risk. Thomas Samaras, an American scientist, reported the risk in the *Bulletin of the World Health Organization* (1992, 70; 2:259). He studied 3,600 baseball players and found a direct relationship between height and life expectancy. "As the men got taller, their average age at death dropped," he says. "It came out to be about one year less life expectancy per inch."

Slap Attack

Men who go bald early in their lives should worry less about their receding youth—and more about their increased chance of a heart attack.

A long-term study of men in Framingham, Massachusetts, found that men who develop "monk's pate" pattern baldness—where hair is lost from the crown on top of the head as well as the front—in middle age, have an increased risk of heart problems.

The researchers report in the *Journal of the American Medical Association* (1993, 269; 8:1035) that they suspect this correlation is linked to dihydrotestosterone (DHT). People with lots of DHT receptors in their scalp tend to go bald early. There are also DHT receptors in other organs, including the heart and liver, where it seems they can also cause problems if they are overstimulated. Scientists at Boston University say that men who develop monk's pate hair loss under the age of fifty-five are particularly at risk.

You could always try to avert this problem by drinking heavily (lawyer's note—don't). Dr. Hugh Rushton, a fellow of Britain's Institute of Trichologists and an authority on hair loss, says alcohol binges protect against baldness. Binge drinkers have livers that are so damaged that they are no longer capable of properly processing the testosterone that lies at the root of the baldness/heart-attack problem.

"If you force a man to drink too much alcohol, it is very unlikely he will lose his hair," claims Dr. Rushton. "How many of the alcoholics you see are ever bald?"

Cardiac Close Shave

Men who do not shave every day are more than three times as likely to suffer a stroke than daily shavers, a twenty-year study indicates. Bristol University researchers asked 2,438 men from Caerphilly, South Wales, how often they needed to lather up. Their susceptibility to heart disease and strokes was then monitored over a twenty-year period.

The study found that those who do not shave every day are also more likely to smoke, less likely to be married, and more likely to do manual work, says the report in the *American Journal of Epidemiology* (2003, 158; 11:1123). But even after adjusting their health risks for these factors, the seldom-shavers were reportedly up to 70 percent more likely to suffer strokes and more likely to die prematurely from any cause.

DISMISSED DISEASES
Some social scourges just seem to disappear

Railway Spine

Along with the new-fangled railways of the 1800s came a whole new-fangled illness: railway spine. People caught up in the era's frequent rail accidents suffered a wide array of symptoms including "obscure affections of the brain and spinal cord." Often these only appeared a long time after the accident.

In many cases such symptoms were seen in patients who had no detectable injury or neurological damage. Others experienced symptoms that were far more serious than one would expect from their modest injuries. Perhaps this was because there were lawyers involved.

Railway spine was usually associated with back pain, other chronic pain, and anxiety—and it was often linked to a compensation claim for damages. The 1923 *Illustrated Family Doctor,* published by the London Household Encyclopaedia, says, "The nervous disorders that may follow a railway collision or any similar accident are usually of hysterical nature. The fact that the patient often recovers very quickly after his claim for compensation has been finally dealt with does not necessarily imply malingering."

When the courts began
to treat sufferers with increasing skepticism, railway
spine largely disappeared

from the medical textbooks. Some experts, however,
say we can thank railway spine—and its psychosomatic
origins—for the birth of American psychotherapy.

Neurasthenia

When neurasthenia appeared in the Victorian era,
thousands of women in America and Europe took to
their beds with a host of vague exhaustion-related symptoms. But around the Second World War, the condition
simply disappeared. George Somerville, the deputy su-
perintendent of London's West Ham Mental Hospital in
1930, described the condition—and the "neurotics" who
suffered it—in *The Hygiene of Life and Safer Motherhood*
manual's special *Personal Supplement*—the section that
women hid in the back of the wardrobe.

"This nervous illness is shown by signs of exhaustion
not only of mind but of body. Most often the woman has
suffered from a state of irritable nerves for some prolonged period before she decides she is really ill. The
symptoms complained of are many. Most characteristi-
cally there is an 'always tired' feeling. All effort, physical
or mental, is painful."

Somerville, not a man given to wild displays of com-
passion, adds: "The neurasthenic woman finds it im-
possible to concentrate, and is unduly self-centred and
excessively concerned with her bodily health. She has an
acute sense of her incapacity and, although she knows

that most of her fears are groundless, she is unable to make the effort to get rid of them. Hence it is of little value to tell the nervous woman to 'buck up' or 'get well.' What is required is to teach her how to make the effort to overcome her troubles.

"The nervous illnesses of women respond well to treatment and the sooner the unhappy victims seek expert advice, the sooner and more completely will they free themselves from the tyranny of 'nerves' and return to their normal health."

What happened to neurasthenia? Some commentators say it got rebranded: critics of myalgic encephalopathy or chronic fatigue syndrome claim it is merely neurasthenia under a new name. The person with myalgic encephalopathy often has disabling fatigue, muscle pain, flu-like malaise, loss of concentration and short-term memory, sensitivity to light and noise, and sometimes depression and mood swings.

Brow ague

This persistent ache behind one eye could prove extremely dangerous, warned English surgeon Johnson Walsham in 1887. No ordinary ache was this; it was "associated with malaria" and could be very painful and be accompanied by twitches. It might also be caused by mouth disease or sinus problems. But failure to remedy it could "unhinge the patient's mind, disposing them towards thoughts of suicide."

An operation could fix it, says Johnson in *Surgery, Its Theory and Practice*. "This is carried out by exposing the nerve above the orbit and raising it on a hook. The hook then draws out the nerve, or it can be rolled over the closed jaws of a pair of forceps. This approach appears singularly successful, as patients rarely return for a further procedure." Hardly surprising really.

Death by Teething

Teething nowadays is considered an inconvenience for babies and parents alike. But historically, the condition has aroused deep fear and apprehension. Hippocrates warned: "Teething children suffer from itching of the gums, fever, convulsions, diarrhoea." And it has even been thought lethal. Fatal teething was listed frequently in early Utah death records.

A physician named Arbuthnot wrote in 1732, "Above one-tenth part of all children die in teething (some of them from gangrene)." As recently as 1979, an English child's death was recorded as "teething convulsions."

The *Western Journal of Medicine* (1991, 155; 6:658) quotes a 1905 American home healthcare book saying, "A very common cause of diseases of the stomach and bowels, and also of convulsions in children, is to be found in the hardening or induration of the gums at the time of teething, and this blunder of nature's ought to be promptly remedied whenever the gums in infants at the time of the first dentition are found to be red, swollen, and hot to the touch."

What actually caused the Utah deaths remains a mystery. From 1847 to 1881, 521 babies' deaths were attributed to teething or related conditions. The number of cases increased gradually each year until 1866, when they jumped significantly. The vast majority of cases occurred from August to December. The level remained relatively high for several more years. Then, almost as quickly, the

number of "teething deaths" fell and virtually disappeared.

Some experts suggest that the actual cause of death
was most likely sudden infant death syndrome (SIDS),
but the average age for "teething deaths" was thirteen
months. Most studies find SIDS usually occurs before six
months.

Floating Kidneys

Doctors don't like to say they don't know what's wrong
with you. So sometimes they will invent an answer. One
of their past creations was the floating kidney. Medics actually believed that patients' vague symptoms were
caused by gravity pulling the kidney down.

The cure? Obvious: fix the kidney in place by putting
a stitch through its wall and hitching it up to some
nearby muscle. In the 1920s and 1930s such operations
were common, averaging twenty a year at Scotland's
Glasgow Royal Infirmary alone. Then quite suddenly it
went out of fashion.

Nymphomania

This was originally a vague term stuck on to any
female sexual desire thought excessive or troublesome. It
was, however, defined as a definite mental illness in
nineteenth-century asylums, where one
cure was to attach leeches to sufferers' vagi-
nas. Historians now consider nymphomania part of a Victorian obsession with
controlling women's self-expression. But "exag-

gerated sexual craving in women" continued to trouble doctors until the end of the twentieth century.

In 1942, the American doctor Edward Podolsky's *Modern Sex Manual* lamented that "For many years the treatment and management of exaggerated sexual craving in women has been a problem which many physicians and psychiatrists have had to face in daily consultation. Frankly there was actually very little that could be done."

Podolsky warned that many women suddenly develop increased sexual desire during menopause. The danger sign was "a sudden increase in weight, which is directly related to the sexual craving." Or perhaps some men suddenly found their obese wives' desires to be excessive.

The doctor thought the sex urge was controlled in women by the pituitary gland at the base of the skull, and that problems began when this became overactive. There was, however, hope, he said: "With startling advances in female hormonology this problem is well on the way toward solution. The new remedy is, strangely enough, the male sex hormone, or testosterone propionate. It is injected once every two days. In most cases, relief is obtained within three weeks or a month. In some cases there is a recurrence of the morbid sex craving."

Alternatives were few: "Mental treatment has been tried, but simply telling a woman to exert some willpower to control her abnormal sex craving is not enough," Podolsky said. The craving could be sublimated, though: "Lecturing, traveling, writing and doing other work which requires physical and emotional expenditure of energy has often been found effective in nullifying unusually strong sexual desire."

Nymphomania was still defined as a sexual deviation in 1951, in America's first official attempt to categorize psychiatric illness: the *Diagnostic and Statistical Manual*

of Mental Disorders. It was still there in 1980, described as
"a psychosexual disorder." Nymphomania only disappeared from the manual in the 1990s.

Nowadays the only female libido "problem," as recently defined by drug companies eager to sell women
sexual stimulants, is female sexual dysfunction, or FSD.
This is characterized by an apparent "lack of desire."
How times change.

OUT OF THE ARC

Nineteenth-century physicians could get a bit too ho-
listic. Many believed that one cause of illness was the
reflex-arc theory. This proposed that every organ in the
body could influence, by reflex, every other organ, no
matter how far away. Toronto University historian Edward Shorter says that because most psychosomatic patients were women, the most popular reflex-arc procedure
was to remove the uterus. The poor patients, with im-
plicit faith in their doctors, suffered gladly, he laments in
his book, *From Paralysis to Fatigue.*

Focal Sepsis

In the early part of the twentieth century, focal sepsis,
or localized infection, usually of the teeth, was blamed
for many illnesses, including rheumatism, gastritis, sclerosis, pernicious anemia, and so on.

The solution: total dental extraction. All your teeth.
Out.

While this was a boon for the dental prosthetics industry, it didn't do much for the poor toothless people di-

agnosed with focal sepsis—whose illnesses were in fact caused by a wide variety of conditions. One by one, the proper causes of the diseases were identified—pernicious anemia, for example, was found to be caused by a deficiency of vitamin B_{12}.

Focal sepsis quietly slunk out of medical textbooks.

Clergyman's Throat

The 1923 *Illustrated Family Doctor,* published by the *London Household Encyclopaedia,* describes this as "A chronic inflammation of the structures at the back of the throat, thus called on account of its being caused to a large extent by an overuse or misuse of the voice. The mucous membrane at the back of the throat is dotted with little dark red elevations varying in size from a pinhead to a pea, or even larger in some cases.

"A visit to a spa possessing laxative waters is often beneficial. The granules at the back of the throat should be destroyed by galvano-cautery or in some other way." Ouch.

Dancing Plague

Mass outbreaks of imagined illnesses did not arrive only with the Industrial Revolution. From the thirteenth to the sixteenth centuries in Europe, large populations became afflicted by the dancing plague—frenzied dancing in which thousands of people became exhausted, often to the point of death.

Dancing plague spread through Holland, Germany, and France over three centuries. It was characterized by an uncontrollable impulse to dance and a morbid love of music, and mostly affected women and poor people. Although it was primarily confined to continental Europe, there was also recorded an outbreak of "the Leaping Ague" in Scotland, and other frenzies in Abyssinia and Madagascar.

At the time, the plague was commonly blamed on demonic possession resulting from invalid baptisms by a corrupt clergy. While its exact cause remains a mystery, it is commonly thought to have been a mass hysterical response to the general misery of life in the grim Middle Ages, with its famines, mass deaths, pestilences, and epidemics. The idea that it was a form of social hysteria is supported by the fact that people only had to see or hear another person dancing to become afflicted themselves.

By the mid-nineteenth century, dancing plague had disappeared. But it was not forgotten. Physicians' suspicion of dancing's anarchic soul reemerged in the journal *Industrial Medical Surgery* (1960; 29:51), where the authors warned that dancing plague had reemerged in the twentieth century in the demonic form of rock 'n' roll.

Perhaps it has not ended there. In 1995, epidemiologists in Newcastle upon Tyne and Fife, Scotland, suggested in *Public Health* (1995; 111:201) that "popular crazes such as breakdancing and raves associated with the drug ecstasy may be the modern-day equivalents. They may be a cultural response to adversity."

Try Suing for These

Defunct occupational illnesses:

Chauffeur's knee
Chimney sweeper's scrotum
Coal miner's nystagmus
Factory fever
Hatter's shakes
Matchmaker's phossy jaw
Painter's colic
Telegrapher's cramp
Woolsorter's disease

Source: "Diseases of Unusual Occupations: An Historical Perspec-
tive," Occupational Medicine: State of the Art Reviews *(1992, 7;
3:369–84).*

SPORT AND LEISURE

Did you really think you'd be safe
at playtime?

Golf-ball Liver

Licking your balls might possibly lower your handicap, but it can also give you hepatitis. Many golfers believe licking the ball can increase its speed in the air. That may be superstitious tosh, but doctors have discovered a definite consequence—golf-ball liver. According to the medical journal *Gut* (1997, 40; 5:687), they discovered the condition in a sixty-five-year-old retired engineer who developed abdominal pain and lethargy while playing golf in Ireland.

The man, who played golf every day, was found after a medical examination to have symptoms of hepatitis, but his doctors could not decide how he acquired the liver disease. Then it emerged that he habitually licked his golf ball clean to make it travel faster, even though signs at the golf course warned of the groundkeepers' widespread use of the weedkiller 2,4-Dichlorophenoxyacetic acid—also known as Agent Orange.

The doctors diagnosed golf-ball liver, caused by the toxic weedkiller he had been swallowing. The patient stopped his golf-ball licking and his symptoms cleared up. But then, skeptical of the medical theory, he started doing it again and landed back at the hospital.

Bolt from the Green

Men are more than four times more likely than women to be struck by lightning, according to *Canadian Geographic* magazine (January 2000). Could this be because they are more likely to play golf?

Golfers are especially at risk because they spend so much time on wide-open courses during the summer, when lightning is most common. The American National Lightning Safety Institute (NLSI) says people on golf courses account for about 5 percent of lightning deaths and injuries each year in the United States.

The most famous incident was during the Western Open golf championship in Chicago on June 27, 1975. The champion player, Lee Trevino, was sitting on the edge of a green by a lake, waiting for a shower to pass, when lightning threw him into the air. He was rushed to the hospital where four burn marks were left on his shoulder where the lightning had left his body. Though his injured back gave him pain for several years, he returned to form.

During the past thirty years, lightning has killed an average of seventy-three people and injured hundreds each year in the United States, says the U.S. National Weather Service. If you are out on the golf course, the NLSI has a simple lightning rule: if you can see it, flee it. The NLSI says to seek shelter when lightning is within six miles of you. God doesn't shout "Fore!"

Penis Substitute?

Men who ride motorcycles to impress women may be in for an unpleasant surprise. French accident-and-emergency-unit researchers have discovered troubling numbers of penile injuries among bikers.

These are caused by riders smacking crotch-first into their gas tanks when their bikes hit an obstacle. This results in hemorrhages, ruptures, and lesions. The doctors from Nice warn in *Injury* (1994, 25; 4:223), "The accident can have after-effects that jeopardise the social and family life of the patients."

Similar damage is reported by doctors in the *Journal of Trauma* (2002, 53; 4:806) who have christened the condition *motor scooter handlebar syndrome.* But there is a positive side. Pathologists from Izumo, Japan, say it can help in the legally important task of finding out who was in control, and who was riding pillion, when both riders die in a crash. Easy, they say in the *American Journal of Forensic Medical Pathology* (1990, 11; 3:190): the pillion rider is the one without the lacerated crotch.

Moving-Goalpost Murder

Look out for that crossbar. Twenty-seven people were killed or injured by falling soccer goalposts between 1979 and 1993 in America alone, reports *Morbidity and Mortality Weekly Report* (1994, 43; 9:153). Sometimes, it's the goalkeeper who needs saving.

Goalkeeper's Finger

Short, married, amateur soccer goalkeeper? Take care of your wedding finger.

The plastic surgery unit at Scotland's Canniesburn Hospital in Glasgow reports in the *Journal of Hand Surgery* (1994, 19; 4:459–60) of three goalkeepers who lost their ring fingers in remarkably similar accidents while setting up their nets.

In each instance, the goalkeeper was trying to attach the nets to the goalposts by jumping up with the netting in his hand while trying to place it over the crossbar hooks. The wedding rings on the goalies' fingers got hooked instead—and there they hung, until they sustained what medical professionals call a degloving injury: the skin of the finger is entirely pulled off and the finger has to be amputated.

The writers warn that amateur soccer goalies are proven to be more prone to the injury than their professional counterparts. Professionals do not have to set up their own nets. More important, all the injured goalies were less than 1.68 m tall—so they had to jump to reach the crossbar. Lessons? Go professional, wear gloves, stay single, and never be a short goalie.

Fun and Games?

The *New England Journal of Medicine* has a habit of publishing physicians' reports of leisure-activity injuries:

There's *Space Invaders wrist.*

Also *cuber's thumb,* caused by obsessive wrestling with a Rubik's Cube.

In a similar vein, there is *GameBox thumb.*

And then there is slot-machine tendonitis—which must be closely related to slot-machine sprain: Richard Nieman, M.D., of the University of California, reveals "an affliction rarely seen by physicians practicing outside of easy driving distance of gambling casinos."

He tells of two patients who complained of painful right shoulders—and no apparent cause—until they said they had both spent the previous weekend on the one-armed bandits. Like many addicts, they had been playing hard and fast.

"Reproduction of the movement required to play slot machines produced excruciating pain," Nieman says in the *New England Journal of Medicine* (1981, 304; 22:1368). Steroids could be injected to relieve the pain but, he writes, "continued trauma after steroid therapy may result in rupture of the tendon." His solution: "Rest—or win a jackpot early."

SCUBA-DIVING DEMENTIA

If you have joined the craze for amateur scuba diving, then be wary. It may cause bends-type brain injuries without anyone even noticing.

Neuroradiologists who studied fifty experienced amateur divers for a *Lancet* report (1995, 345; 8962:1403) found that they had eight times the number of small brain injuries compared with counterparts who engaged in other sports. While the individual injuries to blood vessels in the brain were not significant, they could have a cumulative effect, the report says.

The German researchers say that the injuries, which can be caused by getting the classic diver's bends by resurfacing too quickly and getting nitrogen bubbles in the blood, have been found to cause depression, memory loss, and lower IQ in professional divers.

Bicyclist's Vulva

Mind that vicious cycle: Belgian doctors warn that active women riders can develop this feminine form of saddle-soreness. They report in the *British Medical Journal* (2002, 325; 7356:138) the cases of six women, from ages twenty-one to thirty-eight, who suffered a one-sided swelling of their labia after spending several years cycling on average 462.5 km a week—which in any normal terms could be considered excessive.

It was not the fault of the type of shorts worn, or the cleanliness of each woman's perineum (that bit between front bottom and back bottom), which the doctors, based at Brugmann University Hospital, Brussels, said were all "optimum." But all six women regularly had saddle-related rashes and chronic inflammation of the "saddle area," and five had scars, perineal chafing, and nodules.

Cycling seems to damage the lymphatic system—the body's mechanism for moving fluid around—in the upper thighs, the doctors warn. They conclude that this had caused the women's swellings. They suggest that bikers put their feet up when resting, to aid lymphatic drainage.

The Victorians may have discovered this condition first. The Cycle Touring Club of Great Britain in the late 1800s refused to allow women's racing on grounds of female physiology for several decades.

Pedaller's Penis

Men can be at risk from biking as well. Doctors in Trondheim, Norway, studied 260 male cycle racers after a competition that spanned 540 km, and found many suffered embarrassing problems caused by nerve entrapment. The cyclists developed the male anatomical equivalent of a slow puncture.

Thirteen percent of them suffered impotence for at least a week after the race and 21 percent suffered cycling-related penile numbness. In some cyclists, the symptoms lasted for up to eight months, the researchers report in *Acta Neurology Scandinavia* (1997, 95; 4:233).

Pushbike Prostate

The cycle of misery continues: Kevin O'Brien of the Southern California Permanente Medical Group reports how three men turned up at his practice in the space of a month with problems peeing—an abrupt need to go, or dribbling, feeble wee—all common symptoms of prostate trouble. But no, instead it was pushbike prostate.

"Each patient was able to relate the onset of symptoms either to the purchase of a ten-speed bicycle or an exercise bike," he says. The patients were warned of the danger of putting all their weight on their perineum—that is, sitting on a thin bike saddle. The doctor reports that "voiding habits returned to normal after either discontinuation of cycling or modification of the seat."

But how many men, Dr. O'Brien wonders in the *New England Journal of Medicine* (May 28, 1981), have been

subjected to risky prostate surgery when all they needed
was to get off their bikes?

Unicyclist's Sciatica

In light of this, it is no surprise to learn of unicyclist's
sciatica—caused by the rider putting all of his or her
weight upon the perineum. This was reported by Steven
Gold of the Boston University School of Medicine.

Symptoms include moderate nerve pain down the
buttocks and thighs, and a burning sensation upon peeing. "It is evident that the hazards of unicycle riding go
beyond the obvious orthopedic considerations (e.g., a
broken neck)," he says in the *New England Journal of
Medicine* (1981, 305; 4:231).

Slam-Dunk Death

A simple game of garage-wall basketball could end in
injury or worse. The Royal Australian Institute of Archi-
tects has warned of the dangers of home basketball hoops
after three deaths. The problem? It's the modern craze for
slam-dunking.

Household walls are not built to take the force of a
well-slammed Aussie dunk, where you swing on the hoop
and score mightily. Hapless backyard ballplayers are causing walls to collapse, bringing tons of lethal masonry
down on top of them, warn the experts in Queensland's
Sunday Mail (February 23, 2003).

Snowmobiler's Hematuria

Winter sports fan? You risk a worrisome condition if
you insist on racing around with a full bladder, warns the
Canadian Medical Association Journal (2003, 168; 6:670).
It reports a case of hematuria—that's passing urine with
lots of blood in it—in March 1983, after a patient was
examined for mystery symptoms that were not explained
by the usual diagnoses of sexual infection, or prostate or
abdominal trouble.

Then the patient revealed he was an avid snowmobiler,
and his doctor, Malvinder Parmar (who earlier brought
us Telephone Stroke, see page 5), decided that this was
the cause of the patient's troubles. He says the "repetitive
impact of the man's partially filled bladder against the
bladder base during each thrust caused bladder irritation,
leading to transient gross haematuria."

Parmar speculates that "Because snowmobiling is not
a common recreational activity, this association may be
under-recognized."

Fairground Stroke

Roller coasters can blow your mind. The French doctor Valerie Biousse and colleagues tell of a thirty-one-
year-old female dance teacher who suffered a mild stroke
caused by damage to her left vertebral artery.

She had no history of troubles before admitting herself
to l'Hopital Saint-Antoine, Paris, but said her symptoms
first appeared two days after going on the Space Moun-
tain loop-the-loop roller coaster in Disneyland Paris. "The

delay of forty-eight hours between the onset of pain and the ride on the roller coaster makes it likely that the roller coaster was responsible," says the report in the *Lancet* (1995, 346; 8977:767). Vertebral artery damage "is a frequent cause of stroke in young adults," it adds.

"They are often associated with indirect trauma or torsion of the neck," says Biousse. "The acceleration and abrupt changes of direction on the roller coaster might have induced uncontrolled rotation of the head . . . as observed in some car-crash casualties."

That might sound like an isolated case, but medics are eager to report that it's not all fun at the fair. Minneapolis doctors at the Hennepin County Medical Center report in the *Annals of Emergency Medicine* (2002, 39; 1:65) that between 1979 and 1999, roller coaster rides have been blamed in America for four cases of brain bruising, six burst arteries, three hemorrhages, and one stroke.

ROLLERBLINDNESS

Amusement park rides can make you go temporarily blind, too. Ophthalmologists at the Manchester Royal Eye Hospital, England, report how a short period of intensive roller coaster rides left a nineteen-year-old woman with reduced vision in one eye. They found damage to an artery in her retina, but were happy to report in the *American Journal of Ophthalmology* (2000, 130; 4:527) that her focus returned "after a period of avoidance of roller coaster rides."

Roller-Coaster Love

Those are not the only dangers of thrill-a-minute rides. They can also send you blindly in love, by making you become amorously fixated on complete strangers. This warning on the dangers of inappropriate sexual liaisons caused by roller coasters comes courtesy of Texan psychologists at Austin University, who experimented on passers-by as they were about to get on or off the ride.

They showed the participants a photograph of an average-looking member of the opposite sex and asked them to rate the pictured person's attractiveness and date-worthiness. People riding the roller coaster alone were far more likely to think the person in the photograph sexy after they had finished the ride than before they got on it, the researchers say in the *Archives of Sexual Behaviour* (2003, 32; 6:537).

Why? The shrinks say that it is evidence of "excitation transfer" theory, where people are more likely to be romantically aroused in thrilling or perilous circumstances. We see it happen in adventure films all the time—but you really should be very careful about falling in love with anyone you meet at an amusement park. "This is my new girlfriend. She has a beautiful personality, underneath that beard."

LETHAL STRIKEOUT

Strike one: young athletes, be wary—you are at risk of instant sudden death caused by getting smacked so hard in the chest that it stops your heart. Being struck by a baseball traveling at 40 mph is particularly deadly, reports *Progress in Biophysical Molecular Biology* (2003, 82; 1–3:175).

The impact forces the heart to go into ventricular fibrillation, causing a "significant percentage of deaths on the athletics field," say cardiac experts at Tufts University School of Medicine, Boston. They say that the medical name for this lethal condition is *commotio cordis,* and add, "Sudden death is instantaneous or preceded by several seconds of light-headedness after the chest-wall blow."

The scientists fired baseballs at a hapless young pig and discovered that any ball traveling at 30 mph or more could cause lethal heart trouble. They concluded that 40 mph is the most lethal speed. Any faster or slower was significantly less dangerous.

Two, Four, Six, Eight: Cheerleading Can Devastate

Few sporting activities sound less perilous than prancing around with a pair of pom-poms and a short skirt— but even cheerleading can cause "catastrophic injuries."

Cheerleaders have a five-times higher chance of injury than less showy high-school girls, say North Carolina University orthopods. Their worst accidents are reported to the National Center for Catastrophic Sports Injury Research, which says cheerleading is behind more than half of all sport-related injuries resulting in death or hospitalization.

A study of twenty-nine of the incidents recorded at the Center over a decade shows the easiest way to get severely

hurt is to try building a human pyramid or
performing a "basket toss," where one cheer-
leader is thrown into the air—but not always
caught.

Catastrophic accidents include seventeen se-
vere head injuries, resulting in thirteen skull fractures and
two deaths; three damaged spinal cords; nine broken
necks; and major ligament injuries, say doctors in the
American Journal of Sports Medicine (2003, 31; 6:881).

Go ambulance!

Scrum Strep

Be careful who you headbutt, maul, or grapple in
manly contact sports. You could get a nasty infection. Dr.
John Dorman, student campus medic at America's Stanford University, discovered a new ball-playing peril—
what he calls scrum strep.

This is caused by a bacterial infection of the skin being
passed from one player to another when they thud together.

He tells in the *New England Journal of Medicine* (1981,
305; 8:467) of a case in which a young man came to his
clinic with a streptococcus infection of cuts on his thigh.
The lad went off to play in a local rugby tornament and,
three days later, three more men showed up with the
same streptococcus strain infecting their skin and throats.
A few quick questions established that they had all been
in the same scrimmage together. Similar outbreaks have
occurred involving herpes in wrestlers in 1964, and
among rugby players ten years later.

Lifeguard Lung

So you fancy being a whistle-wielding wow in a *Baywatch* bathing suit? Perhaps you might change your mind if you knew the increased risk of contracting nasty lung infections.

Researchers studying outbreaks of lung disease at pools in Colorado discovered thirty-three lifeguards had lung damage due to infections. The longer the victims had worked as lifeguards, and the longer they worked each day at poolside, the greater their chance of illness.

The study, headed by C. S. Rose of the National Jewish Medical and Research Center, in Denver, found that lifeguards faced up to five-times greater risk if they worked at a pool with a water-spray feature.

These sprays increase the quantity of toxic particles in the air by eight times, the study found. Improving the pools' ventilation systems didn't help either, the scientists report in the *American Journal of Public Health* (1998, 88; 12:1795). Stopping people peeing in the water might, though.

Stranger Than Friction

If the water spray doesn't get you, perhaps the slide will. Experts at the University of Cincinnati medical college's dermatology department report how they were asked to treat a twenty-nine-year-old man complaining of mysterious symmetrical patches on the back of both calves. The traumatized skin looked remarkably like alopecia.

The doctors questioned the man and found that he had spent most of the previous day playing on the water slides at a leisure park. Hence, the big grazed areas on his legs.

He was apparently not smart enough to make the link himself—but at least he enabled the doctors to report the world's first case of *water-slide alopecia* in the skin journal, *Cutis* (2001, 67; 5:399), along with a warning of the dangers of sports-related friction.

Whirlpool Weirdness

Even relaxing in the tub can have its traumas. So beware of whirlpool baths if you have blood pressure or kidney problems. German doctors report the sad case of a thirty-six-year-old man whose kidney was left bruised and bleeding after a vigorous session sitting in front of the bath's water jets.

People who have hypertension or are on anticlotting drugs should be particularly careful because the powerful jets can cause hemorrhaging in vulnerable bathers, warn doctors from the Charite Hospital at Berlin's Humboldt University in a letter to the *Lancet* (February 7, 2003).

Those water jets can also pump you full of dangerous amounts of air if you sit with your orifices too close to them. Radiologists at Washington University's medical school tell of a healthy young woman they examined complaining of severe stomach pains. They discovered she was suffering from extensive pneumoperitoneum— air in the abdominal cavity, a spot where air should not be (see Inflatable Woman Warning, page 28). They report in *Emergency Radiology* (2004, 10; 5:259) that the cause remained a mystery until they discovered she got a lot of pleasure sitting in front of the jets in her whirlpool bath.

A similar case of a woman spending too much time straddling whirlpool water jets was described by British surgeons four years earlier in the *Annals of the Royal College of Surgeons of England* (2000, 82; 5:350). They thought that the problem was previously unheard-of. Perhaps more women enjoy this risky practice than doctors think.

Water-Skier's Enema

Doctors at State University of New York are worried about waterskiing. They say that if you are a woman water-skier and suffer a high-speed fall, you risk getting filled up with harmful torrents of liquid.

They say the problem occurs "when a victim lands on the water at high speed with a cranio-rectal angle of about 120 degrees and the legs abducted" (that means lying back with your feet wide apart). Water is then forced at high pressure into any convenient female orifice.

That can cause hydrosalpinx—an accumulation of watery liquid in the fallopian tubes that is more normally associated with pelvic inflammatory disease. The doctors also say it can cause peritonitis—infection of the abdomen, which can require hospitalization.

The team reports in the *New England Journal of Medicine* (1980, 302; 22:1264) that women's rectums also often get filled up with water. In these patients the doctors observed "sudden onset of crampy abdominal pain followed by intense desire to defecate." They warn, however, "The intense post-traumatic urge to defecate must be respected, and boat owners should carefully question anyone whom they suspect of having waterskier's enema before allowing them back in the boat."

Water-Skier Seer Syndrome

It might seem rather fun to watch a water-skier lose control, but watch out for water-skier seer syndrome, discovered by doctors at Massachusetts General Hospital. They say that people looking back out of the speedboat at the water-skier don't notice when their boat is about to hit a large wave or wake—so they get thrown over the side.

"The boat driver, as a reflex response, turns the boat away from the side of the fall, raising the stern of the boat and driving the propeller over the fallen passenger," they tell the *New England Journal of Medicine* (1979, 300; 15:865). "In three cases, the patients sustained varying degrees of lacerating injuries to the face and upper extremities, which required emergency care and reconstructive surgery."

Surfer's Ear

More board-related havoc is caused by surfer's ear, which is not restricted to surfers. It can afflict anyone who spends time in cold coastal water. It causes lesions in the ear canal, and can block it by up to 90 percent. Understandably, sufferers complain that their ear feels stopped up. Surgery is sometimes necessary, warns the journal *Otolaryngology Head and Neck Surgery* (2002, 126; 5:499).

RUNNING INTO TROUBLE

Runners aren't immune from strange injuries either. Hazards include penile frostbite (*New England Journal of Medicine,* 1997, 296; 3:178)—so think twice before running at night in winter, commando-style, while wearing thin shorts. Up top, there's trouble with jogger's nipple (bleeding nips caused by abrasive clothes).

Swiss researchers warn joggers in the *Schweiz Medizinische Wochenschrift* (1986, 116; 35:1189) that "collisions with vehicles and injuries by buzzards are further possible incidents to be reckoned with occasionally." Now there's something you hadn't prepared for.

Then there is runner's trot—bloating, diarrhea, and flatulence experienced by long-distance runners bouncing their innards about, as revealed in the *Journal of the American Medical Association* (1980, 243; 17:1743).

Sharon Stone Syndrome

Don't try getting fit rapidly if you are over forty. The *Independent* newspaper (November 26, 2001) reports how doctors in California applied to the American Medical Association to register Sharon Stone syndrome in honor of the film star who, at the age of forty-three, was unfortunate enough to suffer a mild stroke while training for a three-mile charity run.

Researchers at Ohio State University claim there has been a massive increase in heart attacks and strokes among the young middle-ageds. The scientists say that thousands of fortysomethings are being killed by exercise as they try to recapture the muscle tone of their youth.

Spot-Kick Killers

Keep a defibrillator handy by the couch next
time you watch international soccer. Heart
attacks on British couches increased by a
quarter when England lost to Argentina in a
televised penalty shoot-out in the 1988
World Cup, say researchers at the universities
of Bristol and Birmingham in the *British
Medical Journal* (2002, 325; 7378:1439).

Risk of admission to the hospital for heart
attack increased by 25 percent on June 30, 1998—
the day of the shoot-out to decide a drawn game—and
on the following two days. No increase in hospital admissions occurred on the previous England match days
in that World Cup.

The researchers blame viewers' stress and conclude that,
aside from questions of sporting fairness, the lottery of the
penalty shoot-out should be abandoned on health grounds.

Instrument Injuries

Music can soothe the troubled soul, but it might not
do much for your health if you are a classical player, according to a study of performers' music-related problems
at a hand-surgery practice. The study of 167 patients
from ages nine to eighty-three found muscle-tendon
strains were the most common problem, occurring prin-
cipally among pianists, violinists, guitarists, and reed in-
strumentalists.

The practice workers discovered (*Medical Problems of
Performing Artists* [2002; 17:135]):

Pianists: 55 percent strains, 17 percent inflammatory conditions, 13 percent nerve problems

Violinists and viola players: 64 percent strains, 7 percent inflammatory conditions

Guitarists: 37.5 percent strains, 22 percent inflammatory conditions, 16 percent nerve problems

Flautists: 25 percent strains, 45 percent inflammatory conditions

Percussionists: 36 percent strains, 36 percent inflammatory conditions.

Art Attacks

Gospel concerts could take you closer to heaven than you expected. Your chances of needing medical help at a musical event depend on the type of music you listen to, says the journal *Academic Emergency Medicine* (1999, 6; 3:202).

Its survey of concert-emergency statistics in America found:

- Highest likelihood of medical emergency: gospel

- Lowest likelihood of medical emergency: rhythm and blues

- Highest likelihood of audience members having heart problems: classical

- Concert with the highest single-day record for medical emergencies: grunge

Reality check: the journal also points out that your chance of needing medical aid at any type of concert is about one in thirty thousand.

When the Fat Lady Sings

Suicide expert Stephen Stack says your chances of suicide are raised if you enjoy listening to operas. The Wayne State University researcher argues in *Death Studies* (2002, 26; 5:431) that opera buffs see so many performances where everyone onstage kills themselves at the end, that they are precisely 2.37 times more open to the idea of copying their example.

He calls this the *Madame Butterfly effect,* and looked to see if it also works in blues fans, who spend so much time listening to unhappy music. He found no direct link, but concluded that listening to Blind Lemon Jefferson and Robert Johnson is more likely to make you reject religion. "And low religiosity is the biggest risk factor for considering suicide," he says.

It Tolls for Thee

Now surely you can't get much safer than bell ringing. However . . . a review of six years' worth of the campanologists' magazine, *Ringing World,* and a survey of twenty operational bell towers has revealed that a disturbing number of bell ringers end up getting tolled off. A total of seventy-nine accidents resulted in ringers getting injured—and in some cases even killed, say doctors at England's Leicester Royal Infirmary in the *British Medical Journal* (1990, 301; 6766:415).

LIVE LONG AND PROSPER

So just how do you cheat the Reaper?

The planet's longest-living people are not necessarily the world's most healthy ones. Mary Dorothy Christian, who was 113 years old and the United States' oldest person when she died in 2003, was a junk-food fiend. Kentucky Fried Chicken and Hostess Twinkies were among Christian's favorites right up until she died.

Sek Yi, a Cambodian tiger hunter said to be the world's oldest man when he died at reportedly 122 years, attributed his longevity and that of his 108-year-old wife, Long Ouk, to smoking and the power of prayer. "When I was young I used to chew betel, but people made fun of me, saying I was like a woman, so I took up smoking," he revealed.

The man confirmed by the *Guinness World Records* as the world's oldest human being ever, Shigechiyo Izumi of Japan, lived to be 120. His favorite drink was an alcoholic beverage called Shochu, which is distilled from barley.

So how do you stay alive, if it is not entirely about being medically healthy? The December 2003 issue of the *Mayo Clinic Women's HealthSource* offers these tips:

- Have a positive attitude.

- Eat well.

- Limit your alcohol consumption. Alcohol's effects are magnified with age.

- Stop smoking.

- Stay physically active.

- Reduce stress by controlling how you react to stressful situations.

- Keep your brain in shape. Lifelong learning is important.

- Keep your social bonds strong. Having a dependable group of friends and family is one of the most reliable predictors of longevity.

- Nurture your spirituality.

- Plan your finances for the future.

Or there's the moral view. From 1921 until 1995, Lewis Terman followed the lives of 1,528 children in California who had been marked for having high IQs. By 1995, half of them were dead. But the study in *Science* (1995; 267:1269) concluded that bright children, especially boys, will live longer if they are prudent, conscientious, truthful, and free from vanity.

Thus it seems that, in spite of the best efforts of today's global health-and-hypochondria industry to keep us fretting over a daily diet of scare stories, strange studies, and silly science, our best hope for enjoying long life and happy health still lies in the old wisdom of simple good living, taking everything in moderation, and trusting to Lady Luck.

So now you know. Well . . . probably. Possibly. Maybe. Perhaps.

INDEX